Psychiatry

Psychiatry

The Science of Lies

Thomas Szasz

Syracuse University Press

Syracuse University Press
Syracuse, New York 13244-5290
Copyright © 2008 by Thomas Szasz

All Rights Reserved

First Edition 2008

10   11   12   13   14   15   6   5   4   3   2

The paper used in this publication meets the minimum requirements of
American National Standard for Information Sciences—Permanence of
Paper for Printed Library Materials, ANSI Z39.48–1984.∞™

For a listing of books published and distributed by Syracuse University Press,
visit our Web site at SyracuseUniversityPress.syr.edu.

ISBN-13: 978-0-8156-0910-0   ISBN-10: 0-8156-0910-8

Library of Congress Cataloging-in-Publication Data

Szasz, Thomas Stephen, 1920–
Psychiatry : the science of lies / Thomas Szasz. — 1st ed.
p. ; cm.
Includes bibliographical references and index.
ISBN-13: 978-0-8156-0910-0 (cloth : alk. paper)
ISBN-10: 0-8156-0910-8 (cloth : alk. paper)   1. Psychiatry—Philosophy.
2. Psychology, Pathological.   3. Mental health—Philosophy.   4. Malingering.   I. Title.
[DNLM: 1. Psychiatry—trends.   2. Attitude to Health.   3. Deception.
4. Malingering. WM 100 S996p 2008]
RC437.5S925 2008
616.89—dc22
2008017999

Manufactured in the United States of America

Truth is mighty and will prevail. There is nothing the matter with this, except that it ain't so.

—Mark Twain (1835–1910), *Notebook* (1898)

Thomas Szasz is a professor emeritus of psychiatry at the State University of New York Upstate Medical University in Syracuse. The author of more than six hundred articles and thirty-two books, he is widely recognized as the leading critic of the coercive interventions employed by the psychiatric establishment.

Contents

Preface

[In the science of politics,] it is inconceivable that telling the truth can ever become more profitable than telling lies.
—Antoine-Augustin Cournot (1801–1877), quoted in *Syphilis, Puritanism, and Witch Hunts: Historical Explanation in the Light of Medicine and Psychoanalysis with a Forecast about AIDS*, by S. Andreski

The widespread belief that the scientist's job is to reveal the secrets of nature is erroneous. Nature has no secrets; only persons do.

Secrecy implies agency, absent in nature. "Nature," observed Thomas Carlyle (1795–1881), "admits no lie."[1] Nature neither lies nor tells the truth. It has no secrets: "secrets" is the name we give to *our* ignorance of its workings. Because nature is not an agent, many of its workings can be understood by observation, reasoning, experiment, measurement, calculation, and truth-telling, the basic methods of science. Deception and divination are powerless to advance our understanding of natural phenomena; indeed, they preempt and prevent such understanding.

The human "sciences" are not merely unlike the physical sciences; they are, in many ways, opposites. Whereas nature neither lies nor tells the truth, persons habitually do both. This is why deception is a useful tool for persons such as detectives whose job is to ferret out other people's secrets; why deception is a useful tool also for so-called experts—such as psychiatrists, psychologists, and politicians—whose ostensible job is to explain and predict certain human behaviors, especially behaviors some people consider dangerous or undesirable; and why such experts habitually deceive others and themselves.

The integrity of the natural scientific enterprise depends on truth-seeking and truth-speaking by individuals engaged in activities we call "scientific," and on the scientific community's commitment to expose and reject errone-ous explanations and false "facts." In contrast, the stability of religions and the ersatz faiths of psychiatry and the so-called behavioral sciences depends on the loyalty of its practitioners to established doctrines and institutions and the rejection of truth-telling as injurious to the welfare of the group that rests on it. Revealingly, we call revelations of the "secrets" of nature "discoveries" but call revelations of the secrets of powerful persons and institutions "exposés."

Psychiatry—a term I use here to include psychoanalysis, psychology, and all the so-called mental health professions—is one the most important institutions of modern societies. The institution rests squarely on the pos-tulate-proposition that "mental illness is an illness like any other illness." That proposition is a lie. This lie is what makes malingering—the faking of disease—the great secret of psychiatry: a popular understanding that fak-ing illness is a form of deception (and often self-deception) would destroy psychiatry. In this book I try to advance such understanding, and the con-structive destruction it entails, by expanding on my thesis, first propounded more than a half century ago: the idea of mental illness and the apparatus of modern psychiatry as a medical specialty rest on the successful medicaliza-tion of malingering—that is, on the popular perception of behaviors called "mental illnesses" as bona fide medical diseases.

Understanding modern psychiatry—the historical forces and the com-plex economic, legal, political, and social principles and practices that sup-port it—requires understanding the epistemology and sociology of faking in general and counterfeiting disease and disability in particular. Where there are fake diseases, there are healthy persons who pretend to be ill and deluded or dishonest doctors who diagnose and treat them. In 1976, protesting the official definition of *psychiatry* as the diagnosis and treatment of mental dis-eases, I proposed this definition:

> The subject matter of psychiatry is neither minds nor mental diseases, but lies . . . [which] begin with the names of the participants in the transac-tion—the designation of one party as "patient" even though he is not ill, and of the other party as "therapist" even though he is not treating any illness. The lies continue with the deceptions that comprise the subject

matter proper of the discipline—the psychiatric "diagnoses," "prognoses," "treatments," and "follow-ups." And they end with the lies that, like shadows, follow ex–mental patients through the rest of their lives—the records of denigrations called "depression," "schizophrenia," or whatnot and of imprisonments called "hospitalization." Accordingly, if we wished to give psychiatry an honest name, we ought to call it "pseudology," or the art and science of lies and lying.[2]

A caricature? Yes. However, a good caricature portrays its subject more accurately than does a flattering portrait, nay self-deluded self-portrait.

Acknowledgments

I am greatly indebted to Anthony Stadlen for his invaluable assistance. I thank also Mira de Vries and Roger Yanow for their careful reading of the manuscript and excellent suggestions, and the staff of library of the Upstate Medical University of the State University of New York in Syracuse for their devoted and generous assistance. As always, my brother George has been a boundless source of information and a sober critic.

Psychiatry

Introduction

The Invention of Psychopathology

Psychopathology: the pathology of the mind; the science of mental disease.
—Oxford English Dictionary

I have dedicated much of my professional life to a critique of the immorality inherent in the practices of the modern misbehavioral sciences (the term is Jacques Barzun's), particularly psychiatry. I say inherent, because deception and coercion are intrinsic to the practices of the mental health professions. The core concept of psychiatry, mental illness qua medical disease, and the profession of psychiatry as a medical specialty based on it, rest on the medicalization of malingering.[1]

The imitation of illness is memorably portrayed by Molière (1622–1673) in his famous comedy *Le malade imaginaire (The Imaginary Invalid)*. As created by Molière, the imaginary invalid, then called a "hypochondriac," is someone who wants to be sick and be treated by others, especially doctors, as if he were sick. Telling Argan, the self-defined patient, that he looks well is considered rude in his household. Molière's invalid confuses religion and medicine—imparting to medicine a sanctity that echoed the mysteries of religion—a confusion then obviously pregnant with comedic possibilities.[2]

Since those days, we in the West have undergone an astonishing cultural-perceptual change of which we seem largely, perhaps wholly, unaware. Today, medical healing is regarded as a form of applied science, the very opposite of faith healing, which is dismissed as hocus-pocus. Mutatis mutandis, the medical profession defines imaginary illnesses as real illnesses, in

1

effect abolishing the notion of pretended illness. Malingering has become a disease "just as real" as melanoma.

Counterfeit art is forgery. Counterfeit testimony is perjury. But counterfeit illness is illness, "mental illness," an illness officially decreed "an illness like any other." The consequences of this policy—economic, legal, medical, moral, philosophical, political, and social—are momentous: counterfeit disability, counterfeit disease, counterfeit doctoring, and the bureaucracies and industries administering, adjudicating, and providing for them make up a substantial part of the national economies of modern Western societies.

According to classic, pathological-scientific criteria, disease is a product manufactured *by the body,* in the same sense that urine is. Diagnosis, in contrast, is a product *manufactured by persons,* in the same sense that works of art are. Charcot and Freud discarded the somatic pathological criterion of disease, destroying the empirical-rational basis for distinguishing real medical disorders of the body (diseases) from fake psychiatric disorders of the "mind" (nondiseases). Modern psychiatry is a gigantic edifice built on the poisoned ruins of this destruction.

Except for a few objectively identifiable brain diseases, such as Alzheimer's disease, there are neither biological or chemical tests nor biopsy or necropsy findings for verifying or falsifying *DSM* diagnoses. It is noteworthy that in 1952, when the American Psychiatric Association (APA) published the first edition of its *Diagnostic and Statistical Manual of Mental Disorders (DSM),* it did not include hysteria in its roster of mental diseases, even though it was the most common psychiatric diagnosis-disease until that time. The term's historical and semantic allusions to women and uteruses were too embarrassing. However, the APA did not declare hysteria to be a nondisease; instead, it renamed it "conversion reaction" and "somatization disorder." Similarly, in 1973, when the APA removed homosexuality from its roster of mental illnesses, it first replaced it with ego-dystonic homosexuality; when that term, too, became an embarrassment, it too was abolished. However, psychiatric researchers lost no time "discovering" a host of new mental maladies, ranging from attention deficit hyperactivity disorder to caffeinism and pathological gambling.

Objective (biological, chemical, physical) tests for diseases are based on the assumption that diseases are somatic phenomena. Accordingly, the claim that mental illnesses are brain diseases is profoundly self-contradictory: a disease of the brain is a brain disease, not a mental disease.

Because there are no objective methods for detecting the presence or establishing the absence of mental diseases, and because psychiatric diagnoses are stigmatizing labels with the potential for causing far-reaching personal injury to the stigmatized person, the "mental patient's" inability to prove his "psychiatric innocence" makes psychiatry one of the greatest dangers to liberty and responsibility in the modern world.

The legal system recognizes the elementary distinction between innocence and guilt. The psychiatric system does not: it proudly rejects the concept of personal responsibility. Crime is a *well-defined act*. Mental illness is an *ill-defined mental state*. Criminal prosecution is defined, and popularly understood, as *adversarial*. Psychiatric treatment, even when forcibly imposed by law, is defined and widely accepted as *nonadversarial*. Those differences, together with the notion of mental illness, are the two great lies and injustices that undergird the psychiatric enterprise.

It is possible to establish that a person accused of a crime is not guilty, that is, has not performed the illegal act attributed to him and is the victim of *malicious prosecution* serving, say, the personal-political ambitions of an unscrupulous district attorney; it is also possible to punish the person responsible for such malicious prosecution.[3] In contrast, it is impossible to establish that a person diagnosed as mentally ill is not mentally ill and is the victim of *malicious psychiatrization* serving, say, the economic-ideological ambitions of the diagnostician; it is not possible to punish the person responsible for the injurious diagnosis that may be *erroneous but, by definition, cannot be malicious*.[4]

In the Anglo-American adversarial legal system, the accused is presumed innocent until proven otherwise, and the onus of proof of guilt is on the accuser. In the psychiatric-inquisitorial "medical" system, this relationship is reversed: the person diagnosed as mentally ill is presumed insane until proven otherwise, and the onus of disproof of insanity is on the (usually powerless) individual incriminated as "insane." A priori, psychiatrists disqualify such claims of "psychiatric innocence" as evidence of the "insane patient's" denial of his illness.[5]

I

One of the most basic mechanisms of deception is imitation, a ubiquitous phenomenon in both the human and the animal worlds. The English language is rich in synonyms for imitation: *bogus, camouflage, chicanery, copy, counterfeit, deception, disguise, dishonesty, duplication, duplicity, fabrication, facsimile, fakery, falsification, forgery, fraud, humbug, identity theft, impersonation, imposture, invention, lie, malingering, mendacity, misrepresentation, perjury, pinchbeck, pirating, plagiarism, pretense, prevarication, sham, simulation, substitute.*[6] Some of the terms we use to describe imitation-as-deception are associated with certain activities and social contexts—for example, *forgery* with art, *perjury* with law, *pinchbeck* with jewelry, *malingering* with medicine. The common denominator among these expressions is the contrast between an original and its copy, the genuine and the imitation.

Incentives for counterfeiting are everywhere. "Practically everything is counterfeited," explains a private investigator engaged in identifying commercial counterfeiters:

> [He] has investigated counterfeit vodka and counterfeit golf balls. He has seen a package of counterfeit prunes. There is counterfeit toothpaste and counterfeit breakfast cereal, and there are counterfeit truck parts (air dryers filled with kitty litter), counterfeit airplane parts (two percent of the parts installed each year), and counterfeit pharmaceuticals (ten percent). . . . Counterfeiting is more profitable than narcotics, and your partners don't kill you. You can import a counterfeit watch from China for a dollar-sixty and sell it on Canal Street for thirty dollars or on the Internet for a hundred and fifty. There ain't no markup like that in narcotics, not ever. And in narcotics if you get caught you go to jail for the rest of your life. If you get caught counterfeiting, you go to jail for three months. Not even.[7]

In this book I consider the elements of the medical situation subject to counterfeiting, such as the impersonation of the sick role by a healthy person (malingering), the impersonation of the healthy role by a sick person (dissimulation), and the impersonation of the role of a physician by a non-physician (quackery).

We must keep in mind that diagnoses are not diseases. In modern societies, everyone may and does make diagnoses: diagnosis making has become democratized, diverse majorities making and unmaking diagnoses. We call that "freedom of speech." However, only one group of persons, called "physicians," is authorized to make official, formally valid, legally consequential diagnoses, which, of course, may be and often are factually false. Also, physicians are authorized to manufacture diagnoses regardless of whether a "condition" so identified is attributable to pathological processes in the body. Finally, officially authenticated diagnoses regularly function as evidence in legal proceedings of all kinds, and their medical validity is rarely if ever questioned.

All of the above is widely known. Nevertheless, to retain their professional credibility, psychiatric historians, like psychiatrists, must believe—or must pretend to believe—that mental illnesses are real in the same sense that cancers are real. As a result, they cannot risk seeing what is in front of their noses. Thus, writing in 1990, Mark S. Micale, a historian of psychiatry, is unable to view hysteria as anything other than a disease entity, hence cannot see that "it" is an example of the virtually limitless human capacity for imitation and wonders why the "symptomatology of the disorder" is so variable:

> The history of hysteria is nothing if not flamboyant. The drama proceeds mainly from the symptomatology of the disorder—rich, colorful, and constantly shifting, personally and culturally, through time. The kaleidoscopic *clinical content of the malady* has made a powerful impression on the popular imagination in the past—and on the scholarly imagination today. The historical idea of hysteria is most likely to bring to mind the gross motor and sensory conversions of the Victorian invalid, the erotic exhibitionism of Charcot's *grandes hystériques,* and Freud's early patients with their abstruse and idiosyncratic neurotica.[8]

To appreciate the wrongheadedness of this medicalized image of counterfeit illness, it will be helpful to briefly review the epistemological foundation of the concept of disease as bodily disorder.

II

The development of the modern cellular-pathological concept of disease was a gradual process, requiring much basic scientific work and the overcoming of medical tradition. The birth of modern medicine as a profession based on empirical science is usually dated to the publication, in 1858, of *Cellular Pathology as Based upon Physiological and Pathological Histology*, by the German pathologist Rudolf Virchow (1821–1902). Emanuel Rubin and John L. Farber, authors of the textbook *Pathology*, state, "Rudolf Virchow, often referred to as the father of modern pathology . . . propos[ed] that the basis of all disease is injury to the smallest living unit of the body, namely, the cell. More than a century later, both clinical and experimental pathology remain rooted in Virchow's cellular pathology." Alvan R. Feinstein, professor of medicine at Yale Medical School, declares, "Virchow's work was magnificent, laying the foundation on which modern histopathology still rests, and demolishing the erroneous doctrine of humoral causes for disease." David M. Reese, an oncologist at the University of California at Los Angeles, writes, "Like Newton's *Principia* two centuries earlier, the work [Virchow's *Die Cellularpathologie*] caused an immediate sensation in Europe. Theories about disease now could be unified under a single rubric, the concept of the cell and its normal and pathological functioning." In this connection, it cannot be overemphasized that whereas a particular pattern of behavior may be the cause or the consequence of a disease, *the behavior, per se, cannot, as a matter of definition, be a disease*. René Leriche (1874–1955), the French founder of modern vascular surgery, aptly observed, "If one wants to define disease it must be dehumanized. . . . In disease, when all is said and done, the least important thing is man."[9]

The definition of disease as cellular pathology is an idea that, as medical historian Erwin H. Ackerknecht puts it, "has dominated biology and pathology up to this very day."[10] Why is this idea so fundamental to the development of medicine as a science? Prior to the cellular-pathological concept of disease, there were many theories of disease, but none was based on empirically verifiable observations or served the interest of advancing knowledge. Instead, each served the interests of its promoter, creating sensational healers and founders of "schools," such as Hippocrates (ca. 460 BC–ca. 377 BC),

Galen (129–ca. 199), and Paracelsus (1493–1541). The somatic pathological definition of disease spelled the end of the old "schools" in medicine and the beginning of medicine as a biological science and as a system of healing based on knowledge rather than belief.

It is or ought to be obvious that having a disease and occupying the patient role are independent variables: not all sick persons are patients, and not all patients are sick.[11] Nevertheless, physicians, politicians, the press, and the public continue to conflate and confuse the two categories.[12] It is a cultural setting conducive to the growth of medicalization: oblivious of the distinction between diagnosis and disease, and between disease and the patient role, the therapeutic state's *furor diagnosticus* rampages triumphantly across the social landscape.

The *Merriam-Webster Online Dictionary* defines *medicalize* as "to view or treat as a medical concern, problem, or disorder" and offers this phrase as illustration: "those who seek to dispose of social problems by *medicalizing* them." The concept rests on the assumption that some phenomena belong in the domain of medicine and some do not, and on an understanding that, unless we agree on *clearly defined criteria that define membership in the class called "disease,"* it is fruitless to debate whether, say, alcoholism or road rage are diseases. Hence, we speak of the medicalization of homelessness and racism but do not speak of the medicalization of malaria or melanoma.

In practice, we must and do draw a line between what counts as medical diagnosis, medical care, or medical service and what does not. Not only must we demarcate disease from nondisease, but we must also distinguish between medicalization from above, by coercion, and medicalization from below, by choice ("forced" on the malingerer by his circumstances). Not by coincidence, these strategies match psychiatry's two paradigmatic legal-social functions: civil commitment–social control and the insanity defense–excuse making.

Medicalization is an aspect of secularization, the therapeutic state (the alliance of medicine and the state) replacing the theological state (the alliance of church and state). Certain behaviors traditionally classified as sins are redefined as sicknesses, justifying their coercive "treatment." As a result, (1) "patients" are deprived of liberty and punished in the name of health; (2) physician-agents of the state assume the task of showing "mercy" toward certain groups of persons—formerly homosexuals, today illegal drug users—by using psychiatric diagnoses to protect them from criminal penalties;[13] and (3) psychiatrists who bootleg certain basic but ambivalently held human values—access to abortion in the past, to marijuana today—are mistakenly perceived as compassionate "humanists" and "therapists."[14]

For example, historian Paul Lerner, in his recent book *Hysterical Men: War, Psychiatry, and the Politics of Trauma in Germany, 1890–1930,* asserts that medicalization is "an inexorable intertwining of healing and medical control" and boldly declares, "Increased psychiatric power and control *saved* thousands of [hysterical] men—including those suspected of malingering—from both severe military punishment and the dangers of the front."[15] This rationalization ignores that, as a matter of public policy and law, replacing criminal sanctions with psychiatric sanctions has far-reaching unintended consequences.[16]

The more apparent it is that, on balance, the medicalization of everyday life harms rather than helps its alleged beneficiaries, the more eagerly psychiatric saviors embrace this medical-statist tactic. Dissenting voices are few and are ignored. One such voice belonged to the late Jonas Robitscher (1920–1981), professor of psychiatry at Emory University in Atlanta. He wrote:

> Following the dissemination of Freudian theory, many conditions that psychiatrists had not previously taken seriously or that they had thought represented malingering were now dignified and given the status of real illnesses. . . . So the incorporation of Freudian thought into medical practice increased the scope of psychiatry in a number of ways. . . . The psychiatrist had received from Freud a new kind of power, different from, and greater than, any he had wielded before. Psychiatrists and psychologists could now claim to understand what was going on in the unconscious.[17]

Ironically, technological advances in medicine, combined with the conflation of the concepts of disease and the patient role, facilitate not only medicalization but also confusion between creating diagnoses and discovering diseases. As a result, when behaviors categorized as diseases are declassified or demedicalized—as happened with homosexuality—science writers, journalists, and the public are easily persuaded by the stakeholders in medicalization that demedicalization, like medicalization, is a product of scientific

progress and moral enlightenment, and not the product of a powe
between interest groups.

Medicalization is not a new phenomenon. Wherever diseased or disabled persons receive care or are excused from certain obligations, the scene
is set for nondiseased and nondisabled individuals to pretend that they
are diseased or disabled. This situation is an example of "medicalization
from below," from powerlessness, for the benefit of the self-defined patient.
"Medicalization from above," the attribution of disease to another—to
control, punish, and disable a person by treating him as a patient, in the
guise of protecting him—is a more recent development, associated with the
birth of psychiatry and psychoanalysis, exemplified by Charcot's classification of "hysteria" as a neurological illness, Krafft-Ebing's "discovery" that
(certain) sex crimes are diseases, and Freud's fabrication of "neuroses" as
"psychogenic" diseases.

Although the process of secularization and medicalization cannot be
attributed to any one individual, it is useful to focus on certain psychiatrists
who were especially influential in fostering the process. One such person was
Baron Richard von Krafft-Ebing (1840–1902), a contemporary of Charcot
and older colleague of Freud. Krafft-Ebing was a German-born physician
who was a professor of psychiatry, successively, at the Universities of Stras-
bourg, Graz, and Vienna. The work that made him world famous is *Psychopathia Sexualis,* the first edition of which appeared in 1886. Krafft-Ebing
was an early practitioner of the art of transforming, with the aid of Latin and
a medical diploma, behaviors considered sinful into sicknesses.[18] Lawyers,
politicians, and the public embraced this new perspective. Sexology became
a part of medicine and "therapeutic jurisprudence" a part of the theory and
practice of criminology.

To impress the medical character of his work on the profession and
the public, Krafft-Ebing sprinkled his text liberally with Latin, and both
he and his publisher maintained that *Psychopathia Sexualis* was intended
only for medical professionals. In the preface to the first edition, Krafft-
Ebing declares, "The object of this treatise is merely to record the various
psychopathological manifestations of sexual life in man. . . . The physician
finds, perhaps, solace in the fact that he may at times refer those manifestations which offend against our ethical and aesthetical principles to a diseased

condition of the mind or the body." I list, without further comment, some of the diseases Krafft-Ebing identified as "Cerebral Neuroses": "*Anaesthesia* (absence of sexual instinct) . . . *Hyperaesthesia* (increased desire, satyriasis) . . . *Paraesthesia* (perversion of the sexual instinct) . . . *Sadism* (the association of lust and cruelty) . . . *Masochism* is the counterpart of sadism . . . *Fetishism* invests imaginary presentations of separate parts of the body or portions of raiment of the opposite sex . . . with voluptuous sensations."[19]

In the 1890s, Krafft-Ebing succeeded in convincing his medical colleagues that sexual perversions—for example, oral and anal sex—are symptoms of bodily diseases. At the same time, Freud failed to convince them that men, too, could "have hysteria." Why did nineteenth-century physicians believe that hysteria could affect only women? Because it was called "hysteria," a term that derives from the Greek *hystéra,* which means "uterus," and because the less people know what they are talking about, the more likely they are to mistake knowing a term for knowing something about the real world. The great physicist Richard Feynman wisely observed, "You can know the name of a bird in all the languages of the world, but when you're finished, you'll know absolutely nothing whatever about the bird. You'll only know about humans in different places, and what they call the bird. So let's look at the bird and see what it's *doing*—that's what counts. I learned very early the difference between knowing the name of something and knowing something."[20] Mistaking knowing the name of something for knowing something is endemic in journalism, politics, and psychiatry.

III

Disease or disability may result in loss of bodily function, loss of income, loss of opportunity, loss of freedom, and loss of life. In contrast, occupying the sick role, with or without having a disease, may enable its occupant to make excuses, gain privileges, obtain money, secure existential opportunities otherwise denied him, and save his life. Children, old people, prisoners, individuals who are or feel victimized, doctors, lawyers, academics, and many others have powerful existential and economic incentives for counterfeiting illnesses and having both counterfeits and counterfeiters authenticated as genuine. In these circumstances, it is easy to see why, as a practical matter, it is virtually impossible to resist the pressures of disease counterfeiting. It is possible, however, to recognize and understand the phenomenon and refuse to be ensnared by it.

Clearly, there are many circumstances in life in which it is useful to be ill or to be regarded as ill by others. This is what renders counterfeiting illness not merely valuable but virtually indispensable. Who among us has not turned down an unattractive social obligation by pleading illness? Who has not manufactured a "symptom"—for example, insomnia—to obtain a sleeping pill available only by prescription?

A genuine article is distinguished from its counterfeit by its provenance or origin. In the case of a painting by a famous, long-dead artist, its provenance is established by its history, by documents attesting to the identity of former owners, and perhaps by a scientific-technical examination of the composition of the canvas and paints. In the case of a common commercial product, provenance is established by the legal mechanism we call "patent" or "trademark," such as Coca-Cola or Kodak. A patent is a set of exclusive rights granted by the state to a patentee, for a fixed period of time, in exchange for the public disclosure of certain details of a device, method, or process. The patent protects the inventor's property right in the product, that is, his right to prevent others from making, using, or selling the invention. Without such a fixed standard of what counts as an "original," say, Nike sneaker, it would be impossible to distinguish genuine Nike sneakers from good imitations. Although the original and the counterfeit may look alike and be of the same quality, the *legal difference* between them is clear: it is a matter of whether the agent has or has not the right to produce the product and represent it as the "original."[21]

Let us ask the crucial questions once more: What counts as genuine disease? Who has the "right to produce illness"? How do we distinguish real disease from faked disease, literal illness from metaphorical illness? Physicians, as we have seen, are legally authorized to manufacture diagnoses regardless of disease criteria, and the media may assist them in conflating invented diagnoses with imaginary illnesses. But they cannot create or produce diseases.

We use two criteria to distinguish real diseases from fake diseases: one is phenomenological, the other etiological. Phenomenologically, to qualify as a disease, the condition must be objectively identifiable as a *pathoanatomical or pathophysiological* lesion or process—for example, a microbial infection or histologically demonstrated cellular abnormality. Etiologically, the condition must be a *product of impersonal natural forces or processes* or *of physical injury*—for example, a malignant process or bone fracture. These measures are not my idiosyncratic criteria. To the contrary, they are the conventional nineteenth-century pathological criteria of disease, formulated to place diagnosis and treatment on a scientific foundation. It is this foundation that physicians then used to lobby the state to create a medical monopoly restricting the practice of medicine to physicians whose training is attested to, and whose privilege—often erroneously called a "right"—to practice their craft is granted by the state. However, it is not science but the alleged interest of the public that rationalized and justified this restriction. During approximately the same period that medicine acquired an increasingly science-based foundation, so also did many other fields of practical knowledge, such as chemistry and nutrition. Yet neither chemists nor cooks need a license to practice their craft.

The restriction of the role of medical doctor to academically qualified and legally licensed physicians contained certain clear, albeit inexplicit, duties on the parts of both doctors and patients. The honest physician may diagnose disease if, and only if, the sufferer has a bona fide illness; the physician who diagnoses a healthy person as sick is a cheat and a quack. Similarly, the honest patient may assume the sick role if, and only if, he suffers from a real disease; the healthy person who assumes the sick role is a cheat and a malingerer. That, at least, was the theory. In practice, neither party ever abided by these tacit rules. The reasons they didn't are simple, and it is important that they be clearly understood.

The rules I just articulated depend on the materialist-pathological definition of disease that became the gold standard of medicine only during the second half of the nineteenth century. The practice of mad-doctoring, however, had been well established before that time, when medicine was still based on the so-called humoral theory of disease. According to that view, every condition that a doctor or patient called "disease" was, a priori, a material-corporeal, "humoral" abnormality. Everyone believed to be ill was regarded as suffering from a "humoral imbalance." The mad-doctor's principal duty was to incarcerate the patient and attach a diagnostic label to his alleged disease. Curing the madman, like curing any sick patient, required correcting his humoral imbalance. For the most part, prisoner patients were deprived of liberty not because they were ill but because they annoyed others. The diseases attributed to them were rationalizations for their involuntary detention and for the interventions forcibly imposed on them.

From the start, diseases called "mental" were characterized by the *failure* of physicians to find somatic signs or markers for their putative maladies. Disabilities attributable to bodily organs were considered diseases of the body, not the mind. As the nineteenth century progressed and as the study, practice, and teaching of medicine became based increasingly on anatomy and pathology, many physicians realized that mental diseases are not, and could not be, genuine diseases. The first physician to emphasize that the mental patient's alleged illness is a metaphorical, not a literal, illness was Viennese surgeon Baron Ernst von Feuchtersleben (1806–1848).[22]

This admission did not mean, however, that Feuchtersleben wanted to exclude mad-doctoring from medicine or delegitimate mad-doctors as quacks. On the contrary, he wanted to strengthen the legitimacy of both, creating the key term *psychopathology,* denoting a class of "diseases" that affect the mind rather than the body. The *Oxford English Dictionary (OED)* in the epigraph credits Feuchtersleben as being the first person to use the term, in 1847 (the date of publication of *The Principles of Medical Psychology* in English). It was at this time, too, that the term *psychogenic* became a part of the vocabulary of medicine. (The *OED* traces the origin of the term to the 1830s, first used in a nonmedical context.)

IV

Jean-Martin Charcot (1825–1893), Sigmund Freud (1856–1939), and Pierre Janet (1859–1947) all ignored the denominated mental patient's legal status (regardless of how he became transformed from person into patient), assumed that he had a "psychopathological" disorder, and focused on its pathogenesis, that is, on what made the patient sick. Noting that the subjects' "abnormal mental state" lacked a somatic cause, they embraced and popularized the notion of "psychogenesis." "Diseases" formerly called "imaginary" or "self-caused" were renamed "psychogenic diseases" and declared to be just as genuine as real diseases produced by agents external to the self, including the body. *Essential for this process was the deceptive and self-deceptive separation of the abstract noun "mind" as quasi agent from the concrete person as responsible actor.* Malingering was thus transformed into hysteria, hysteria was generalized into neurosis, and neurosis proliferated into the 350 distinct "psychopathological" entities now recognized as "mental disorders" by American psychiatry, American psychology, American medicine, and American law as well as by similar national and international authenticating bodies and health insurance companies.

What materialist medical science gave with one hand, biopsychosocial medical-psychiatric scientism took away with the other. The boundary between genuine diseases and counterfeit diseases, diseases and nondiseases, was breached. The differences between happenings and actions, between material objects manufactured by bodies (urine, inflammation) and immaterial ideas manufactured by persons (thoughts, schizophrenia), were officially abolished. Given carte blanche to counterfeit diseases, agents of the therapeutic state created the disease inflation with which we are familiar. Pari passu, drugs and drug use became politicized, with similarly familiar consequences.[23]

Although there are no mental illnesses, there assuredly are unwanted behaviors and persons. The point is that we mistake behaviors called "mental illnesses" for real illnesses just as we mistake counterfeit one hundred–dollar bills for genuine one hundred–dollar bills. The difference is that counterfeit bills can be exposed as fakes, whereas "mental illnesses" cannot. Indeed, so deep and widespread is the popular faith in fake illnesses as real diseases that persons who deny their medical legitimacy or status are routinely branded as crazies, modern flat-earthers. Even experts inclined to take a skeptical view of psychiatry continue to use the term *mental illness.* Noted historian of psychiatry Roy Porter writes, "It is important to remember that even today we possess no rational consensus upon the nature of mental illness—what it is, what causes it, what will cure it." Nancy Andreasen, one of the best-known American schizophrenia researchers, admits that she does not know what schizophrenia *is:* "Europeans can save American science by helping us figure out who really has schizophrenia or what schizophrenia really is."[24] But there is no "it" that "really is" schizophrenia. Nevertheless, responding to individuals now categorized as schizophrenic *patients* as nonsick *persons* would so dis-order modern societies that any movement in that direction appears to be precluded, at least for the foreseeable future.

Scientific work requires detachment from the tumults and tragedies of everyday life, calm reflection, and brutal honesty. Medical science and medical practice are two very different enterprises. There is good reason that medical science developed at the autopsy table and was based on the study of cadavers, whereas medical practice developed at the bedside of sick individuals and was based on the observation and treatment of suffering persons. There is also good reason that psychiatric pseudoscience developed wherever explanations for baffling behaviors were sought and why psychiatric practice developed in domiciles wherever people with such behaviors were incarcerated, cunningly called "asylums" and "hospitals."

V

Attributing a medical diagnosis to a healthy person does not transform him into a bodily-medically ill person, whereas attributing a psychiatric diagnosis to him does indeed transform him into a mentally-psychiatrically ill person.

A nephrologist may declare Smith to be suffering from uremia. But if Smith does not, in fact, have kidney failure, then the diagnosis will not make him sick. It will make the diagnosis erroneous. In contrast, a psychiatrist may declare Smith to be suffering from schizophrenia. Regardless of Smith's behavior or mental state, the diagnosis will transform him into a "schizophrenic," or at the very least into a "schizophrenic in remission." In medicine diagnoses are not diseases and do not justify incarcerating patients, but in psychiatry diagnoses are mental diseases and (may) justify incarcerating patients. In short, depending on the circumstances, psychiatric diagnoses qua diseases function as exculpations, protecting individuals, or as inculpations, endangering them. Not by coincidence, these effects are the consequences of the psychiatrist's paradigmatic practices—the insanity defense and civil commitment.

Infectious diseases—malaria, tuberculosis, typhoid fever, and others— are the sources of human problems and deaths. Psychiatry rests on attributing all manner of human problems and deaths to a similar impersonal mechanism—illustrated by such false beliefs as that schizophrenia causes crime and depression causes death.

Psychiatry, psychoanalysis, and the mental health professions are the intellectually, morally, and politically toxic side effects of the development of scientific medicine. Still, regardless of evidence or reasoning, most people "believe" in mental illness, claiming that "its" existence is obvious. It is not surprising. People who regularly use God language come to believe in his "existence" (and vice versa), and the belief makes them apprehend God, called "theophany." We regularly use mental illness language and come to believe in its "existence" (and vice versa), and the belief makes us apprehend psychopathology. I call it "psychopathophany."

1 Malingering

> All neurotics are malingerers; they simulate without knowing it, and
> this is their sickness.
>
> —Sigmund Freud, quoted in *Freud as an Expert*
> *Witness: The Discussion of War Neuroses Between Freud*
> *and Wagner-Jauregg,* by Kurt R. Eissler

In 1835, the University of Edinburgh held an essay contest titled "The Best Classification of the Feigned and Factitious Diseases of Soldiers and Seamen, on the Means Used to Simulate or Produce Them, and on the Best Modes of Detecting Impostors." The winner was a medical student named Hector Gavin. In 1843, Dr. Gavin published his essay in a revised and enlarged version.[1]

Gavin's treatise runs to 436 pages and consists of the description of hundreds of complaints, each qualified with the adjective *pretended*. Today, most of this material is of antiquarian interest only. Gavin's introductory comments, however, remain relevant: they remind us that malingering is a ubiquitous phenomenon that occurs among all peoples, has occurred at all times, and was formerly punished as a crime:

> Disease has been simulated in every age and by all classes of society. The monarch, the mendicant, the unhappy slave, the proud warrior, the lofty statesman, even the minister of religion, as well as the condemned malefactor, and "boy creeping like snail unwillingly to school," have sought to disguise their purposes, or to obtain their desires, by feigning mental or bodily infirmities. . . . Those who simulated diseases were formerly punished as forgers; and it appears from history that the Greeks were exceedingly severe against such persons. . . . Malingerers in this service [the Austrian military

17

in the 1830s] are severely punished: sometimes they receive corporal punishment, and at other times they are sentenced to serve for life.[2]

As if anticipating the hundreds of discrete mental illnesses now officially
accredited as medical diseases, Gavin adds, "As diseases are feigned for a
variety of purposes, so the character of the assumed disability is calculated to
suit the occasion."[3] Throughout his treatise, Gavin's attitude toward malingering is hard-nosed: malingerers are fakers and are of interest to doctors
only because they must distinguish them from sick persons.

During the latter half of the nineteenth century—by which time the
scientific revolution in medicine placed the definition of disease on the
solid foundation of empiricism and somatic pathology—physicians began
to regard a certain type of counterfeit illness as a real disease, called it
"hysteria," and relaxed their efforts to locate "it" in the body. Instead, they
focused their attention on managing every kind of personal conduct *they
called "hysteria"* (later, "neurosis" or "mental illness") with medical controls *they called "treatment."* This reinforced and reenergized the old connections between mad-doctoring and law enforcement that, in turn, made
artists and social critics increasingly skeptical about the new "science of
psychiatry," suspecting both its alleged maladies and its supposed cures of
being fraudulent.

An 1846 caricature by Honoré Daumier (1808–1879) is an early example of the commonsense insight into the truth about psychiatry as excuse-
making and social control. The scene is a prison cell. The unkempt prisoner
sits on a cot, his dandified lawyer standing before him. "What really both-
ers me," says the prisoner, "is that I have been accused of twelve robber-
ies." "Twelve of them," replies the lawyer. "So much the better. I will plead
monomania."[4] This joke has since become the everyday reality of our age.

Roughly between 1850 and 1880, malingering became transformed
into hysteria, and psychiatry—increasingly distinct from neurology—
became a popular belief system, a medical-secular religion. Terms such as
imposturing, malingering, and *self-caused disease* fell into disrepute and were
abandoned, and the terminology of hysteria and other counterfeit maladies
was incorporated into the vocabulary of medicine.[5] Modern psychiatry—
with its *Diagnostic and Statistical Manuals* of nonexisting diseases and

their coercive cures—is a monument to quackery on a scale undreamed of in the annals of medicine.[6]

I

In 1853, Robert Brudennel Carter, a British general physician, published a pioneering work, *On the Pathology and Treatment of Hysteria*. Both the title and the contents of the book reflect the newly emerging zeitgeist of medicalization. Actually, the assertively medical ring of Carter's title conceals his doubts about whether the term *hysteria* denotes a real disease: he laments the "inexactness unparalleled in scientific phraseology" of the discourse about hysteria, notes that its "symptoms" range from complaints "referable" to the brain and its coverings to "hypochondriasis . . . [and] simple malingering," and warns about "the evil consequences which so often follow the attempt to give a definite name to an unknown quantity."[7]

Hysteria is a classic example of the error against which John Selden (1584–1654), the celebrated seventeenth-century English jurist and scholar, had vainly warned: "The reason of a thing is not to be inquired after, till you are sure the thing itself be so. We commonly are at, *what's the reason for it?* before we are sure of the thing."[8] The problem is that, in everyday affairs where concepts and categories are often ill-defined or are defined by reference to authorities rather than objective criteria, it is virtually impossible to adhere to Selden's stricture.

In psychiatry especially, it is often virtually impossible to be sure "what a thing itself really is," because "the thing itself" is prejudged by ordinary language.[9] We in the West identify two very different kinds of behaviors as diseases or as symptoms of disease: morally appropriate conduct that looks like a disease (for example, fatigue) and deviant or illegal conduct that society and the law want to control by medical rather than penal sanctions (formerly homosexuality, today homelessness, domestic violence, drug use, suicide).

Carter recognized that hysteria is a two-person phenomenon, that is, the product of communication-collusion between a subject who pretends to be sick and a medical authority who validates the impersonation: "The professional man who has once sanctioned imposture, by sending medicines for the cure of self-produced illness, becomes at once an ally, whose aid is the more important for being unconsciously rendered. . . . Against [hysteria] . . . I should regard all medicines to be absolutely useless and inert. . . . [they] can scarcely fail to exert an injurious moral influence."[10]

Another important figure in the early history of the medicalization of malingering was Ernst von Feuchtersleben. A graduate of the University of Vienna's medical school, Feuchtersleben practiced and taught surgery, was active in educational reform, and was also a respected poet. He is the author of two books on "mental illness." The first, a major treatise, *Lehrbuch der ärtzlichen Seelenkunde* (Textbook of the Medical Cure of Souls), translated as *The Principles of Medical Psychology,* was published in 1835. The second, *Zur Diätetik der Seele,* a slim volume, appeared in two different American editions: one titled *The Dietetics of the Soul* (1838), the other titled *Hygiene of the Mind* (1933).

Feuchtersleben deserves to be better known than he is: he coined the term *psychopathology* and recognized that mental illnesses are not "like other illnesses" but that, unavoidably, they play an important role in the everyday practice of medicine and in the expanding field of "judicial psychology" (forensic psychiatry). In *The Principles of Medical Psychology,* he memorably stated: "The maladies of the spirit *[die Leiden des Geistes]* alone, *in abstracto,* that is, error and sin, can be called diseases of the mind only *per analogiam.* They come not within the jurisdiction of the physician, but that of the teacher or clergyman, who again are called *physicians of the mind [Seelenärzte]* only *per analogiam.* The maladies of the body alone *in abstracto,* for instance, of the brain or nerves, without mental alienation, are not diseases of the mind, but of the body."[11]

II

During the winter of 1885–1886, Sigmund Freud spent about four months in Paris studying the work of the famed neurologist Jean-Martin Charcot. In April, after returning to Vienna, he wrote his first paper on neuropathology/psychiatry, "Report on My Studies in Paris and Berlin" (1886): "In my application for the award of the Travelling Bursary from the University Jubilee Fund for the year 1885–6, I expressed my interest in proceeding to the Hospice de la Salpêtrière in Paris and there continuing my studies in neuropathology. Several factors had contributed to this choice. [One] was the great name of J.-M. Charcot. . . . The French school of neuropathology . . . [has] embarked on new fields of neuropathology, which have not been similarly approached by scientific workers in Germany and Austria."[12]

What were these "new fields of neuropathology" to which Freud alludes? He tells us:

> Charcot used to say that, broadly speaking, *the work of anatomy was finished and that the theory of organic diseases of the nervous system might be said to be complete: what had next to be dealt with was the neuroses*. . . . For many years now his work has been centered almost entirely on the neuroses, and above all on hysteria. . . . In his study of hysteria Charcot started out from the most fully developed cases which he regarded as the perfect types of the disease. . . . By making a scientific study of hypnotism . . . he himself arrived at a kind of theory of hysterical symptomatology. These symptoms *he had the courage to recognize as for the most part real.*[13]

In view of Charcot's lofty position in French medicine and society, his "discovery" of a disease without somatic pathology required chutz-pah, not courage. A subject's complaints/reports, verbal and nonverbal communications/"symptoms" are, by definition, "real." The observer's/physician's interpretation of them is a very different matter. The assertion that they are manifestations of a disease of the central nervous system may be true or false; treating them as such may help or harm the denominated patient, depending on what he wants and irrespective of whether he is sick. Swiss psychiatric historiographer Henri Ellenberger cogently notes, "Neurologists, some of whom remained [Charcot's] admirers *as long as he stayed on the solid ground of neuropathology, deserted him when he shifted to the study of hypnotism and the spectacular experiments with hysterical patients.*"[14]

In his report, Freud writes as if it were self-evident that hysteria is a neuropathological illness. In the 1880s, all disease was, by definition, "somatic," that is, the pathology of organs and tissues. The "mind" is not a bodily organ. The German language does not even have a term for "it."

Freud went to Paris like the Muslim pilgrim goes to Mecca, to reaffirm and strengthen his faith. It is clear from his report that before leaving Vienna for Paris, Freud had decided to give up the study of real diseases and the practice of real medicine and embark on the study of fake diseases and the practice of fake medicine. Commenting on the *grand hypnotisme* (major hypnotism) described by Charcot, Freud writes, "I found to my astonishment that here were occurrences plain before one's eyes, *which it was quite impossible to doubt,* but which were nevertheless strange enough not to be believed unless they were experienced first hand. . . . [T]he whole trend of his mind leads me to suppose that he can find no rest till he has correctly described and classified some phenomenon with which he is concerned, but that *he can sleep quite soundly without having arrived at the physiological explanation of that phenomenon.*"[15]

Here we catch Freud with his hand in the cookie jar, and not for the last time. He calls Charcot's theatrical performances "occurrences plain before one's eyes, *which it was quite impossible to doubt.*" Au contraire. Had Freud known more science, he would have been familiar with the Marquis de Laplace (Pierre-Simon Laplace [1749–1827])—mathematician and astronomer, often dubbed the "French Newton"—who had warned: "Extraordinary claims require extraordinary proof."

Freud was not interested in scientific proof. He was interested in psychological proof, which is no proof at all. At the same time, though he lacked both the knowledge and the temperament for doing real science, he persistently claimed that psychoanalysis is a branch of natural science. Freud was a man of the Enlightenment. Instead of believing in God, he believed in Charcot. The age of medicalization had dawned. Validating fake illness as real illness, psychopathology as neuropathology, Charcot opened the floodgates. Freud proceeded to inundate the world with fake diseases, perverting the epistemology of disease and corrupting the ethics of medicine.

III

It is often said that to successfully deceive another, one must first deceive oneself. German psychiatrist Ernst Kretschmer (1888–1964) cited this adage in relation to the illusory difference between malingering and hysteria: "Should we not much rather conclude: the more honest the conviction of illness, the better the deception—of himself and others? For he deceives the most deceptively who deceives himself as well."[16]

Freud deceived himself by simultaneously maintaining two internally contradictory propositions: that "neurotics" are the victims of real (hetero-genic) *diseases,* hence bona fide medical patients, and that they are moral agents who pretend to be ill by producing fake (autogenic) *symptoms,* hence malingerers.[17] In the *Introductory Lectures on Psychoanalysis* (1915–1917), he condenses this contradiction into a single sentence: "Thus a healthy per-son, too, is virtually a neurotic, but dreams appear to be the only symptoms which he is capable of forming" (Auch der Gesunde ist also virtuell ein Neu-rotiker, aber der Traum scheint das einzige Symptom zu sein, das zu bilden er fähig ist).[18] Note that Freud calls dreams "symptoms" and attributes their genesis and content to the dreamer.[19]

What was Freud's basis for regarding "neurosis" as a real disease rather than a counterfeit disease? Only that Charcot said so. Like Charcot, Freud emphasized that neuroses lacked a neuropathological basis. What, then, was the problem Charcot, Freud, and others called "hysteria" and "treated" as if it were a disease? It was that the medical practitioner often found himself in the presence of a person, usually a young woman, who said she was sick or was said to be sick by a relative or caretaker, but whose medical examina-tion revealed her to be healthy. The physician suspected that the patient was malingering. What was he to do?

Socially, the person called "patient" was considered to be sick before encountering the physician. The physician was expected to validate the sub-ject's disability as owing to disease by diagnosing the illness and treating it. The doctor's most obvious but professionally most incorrect option was to conclude either that the subject malingers or that he, the physician, is unable to find a disease to account for the patient's complaints, and decline to care for her or him. Some physicians did that very thing, ceding the ground to charlatans such as Franz Anton Mesmer (1734–1815) and the hypnotists. The doctor's other option was to conclude that the patient was mentally ill, that she suffered from hysteria. That decision is what Freud and the post-neuropathological psychiatrists made. Thus arose the modern idea of mental illness, the product of the conflation of having a disease and occupying the sick role (voluntarily or involuntarily).

The view that pretending to be mentally ill is itself a form of mental illness became psychiatric dogma during the Second World War. Kurt R.

Eissler (1908–1999), the quasi-official pope of the Freudian faith in the United States, declared: "It can be rightly claimed that malingering is always the sign of a disease often more severe than a neurotic disorder. . . . It is a disease which to diagnose requires particularly keen diagnostic acumen. The diagnosis should never be made but by the psychiatrist."[20] Diagnosing the fatal conceit of the power-mad expert requires no acumen at all.

Now, more than fifty years later, this medicalized concept of malingering is an integral part of the mind-set of every well-trained, right-thinking Western psychiatrist. For example, Phillip J. Resnick, a leading American forensic psychiatrist, speaks about "diagnosing" faked mental illness as if it were a real disease: "Detecting malingered mental illness is considered an advanced psychiatric skill, partly because you must understand thoroughly how genuine psychotic symptoms manifest." Dutch psycholinguist Victor Kuperman recognizes that "malingering or dissimulation presents a fundamental problem *capable of undermining the entire psychiatric enterprise*," and beats a hasty retreat from this dangerous insight by pontificating about "Foucauldian categories [of] folly" and "the *clinical* phenomenology of malingering."[21]

In World War I, soldiers afraid of being killed in battle malingered; psychiatrists who wanted to protect them from being returned to the trenches diagnosed them as having a mental illness (then called "hysteria"). Today, ninety years later, soldiers returning home and afraid of being without "health care coverage" diagnose themselves as having a mental illness (now called "post-traumatic stress disorder [PTSD]"). The soldiers themselves candidly acknowledge this motive. Almost 50 percent of the troops returning from Iraq suffer from post-traumatic stress disorder and depression "because they want to make sure that they continue to get health care coverage once their deployments have ended." The reporter relates this tactic matter-of-factly. Indeed, he titles his story, "In Iraq as in World War II, Soldiers' Wounds Go Well Beyond the Physical," using the word *wound* both literally and metaphorically.[22] The literalization of the metaphor "mental illness" has evolved so far that acknowledging it no longer threatens its status as an "illness like any other." In *The Myth of Mental Illness,* I took this semiotic bull by its metaphorical horns and showed that it was "bull" indeed: there is no mental illness.

In 1960, I coined the term *myth of mental illness* to suggest that the distinction between bodily illness and mental illness rests on a misuse of the term *illness*. When we say that Smith has a mental illness, we misidentify his strategic behavior as a bodily disease (an objectively identifiable physical phenomenon with its origin not directly under human control). If we limit the use of the term *illness* or *disease* to observable biological—anatomical and physiological—phenomena, then, by definition, the term *mental illness* is a metaphor. Mind is not matter, hence mental illness is a figure of speech. The idea of two kinds of diseases, one bodily, the other mental, is an unintended product of the scientific revolution: the imitation of science, called "scientism." *Hysteria, schizophrenia, mental illness,* and *psychopathology* are scientistic, not scientific, terms.

In the past fifty years psychiatry has "progressed." Today, self-diagnosis with mental illness suffices to legitimate the self-diagnoser as a "sick patient" who has insight into his illness and recognizes his need for treatment. Now, the bête noire of psychiatry is his opposite number, the person who lacks insight into his illness, is "treatment resistant," or displays "negative attitudes toward treatment-seeking." From the *International Journal of Eating Disorders* we learn: "Considering that males have negative attitudes toward treatment-seeking and are less likely than females to seek treatment, efforts should be made to increase awareness of eating disorder symptomatology in male adolescents, and future prevention efforts should target male as well as female adolescents."[23]

IV

Some nineteenth-century physicians—notably the famous American neurologist Silas Weir Mitchell (1829–1914), inventor of the legendary "rest cure" named after him—recognized that hysterics were malingerers. Having worked as a physician during the Civil War, he saw a good deal of malingering and understood it for what it was: the rational assumption of the sick role. Confronted with such persons—regardless of whether they were called "hysterics"—he realized that the person who assumes the sick role is not necessarily sick and that hysteria is not a bona fide disease.[24]

Because Mitchell was the son of a prominent Philadelphia physician and was himself a famous physician and man of letters, he possessed the professional and social standing that allowed him to engage in some unorthodox therapeutic methods. Realizing that the problem he was called upon to treat was drama, not disease, Mitchell treated it accordingly. Consulted about a woman believed to be mortally ill, Mitchell dismissed all present in the room and then left himself. "Asked of her chances of survival he answered: 'Yes she will run out of the door in two minutes; I set her sheets on fire.'"[25] Seeing another hysterical woman who claimed to be unable to get out of bed, he "threatened her with rape and commenced to undress. He got to his undergarments when the woman fled the room screaming."[26]

Like Mitchell, Josef Breuer (1842–1925) was a successful physician, financially comfortable, and secure in his medical role. That background, together with his firm footing in medicine, helped him see that hysteria was theater, not medicine. He effortlessly transcended Freud's self-created pseudoscientific metaphorizations. In the concluding part of *Studies in Hysteria,* Breuer declares (in the English translation by James Strachey), "In what follows little mention will be made of the brain and none whatever of molecules. Psychical processes will be dealt with in the language of psychology. . . . If instead of 'idea' we chose to speak of 'excitation of the cortex,' the latter term would only have any meaning for us in so far as we recognized an old friend under the cloak and tacitly reinstated the 'idea.' . . . The substitution of one term for another would seem to be no more than a pointless disguise." In the German original, the last sentence is: "Jene Ersatz der Termini scheint eine zwecklose Maskerade."[27] Faithfully translated, it would read: "That replacement of terms seems a pointless masquerade," which is a more powerful statement than the one conveyed by Strachey's translation. There is no waffling here with "would seem to be," and "masquerade" is stronger than "disguise." Strachey minimized the importance of the sentence, which, in the German, stands at the beginning of a new paragraph, by merging it with the previous paragraph. Breuer continues:

> It is only too easy to fall into the habit of thought which assumes that every substantive has a substance behind it—which gradually comes to regard "consciousness" as standing for some actual thing; and when we have

become accustomed to make use metaphorically of spatial relations, as in the term "sub-consciousness," we find as time goes on that we have actually formed an idea which has lost its metaphorical nature and which we can manipulate easily as though it was real. Our mythology is then complete.

(Allzuleicht verfällt man in die Denkgewohnheit, hinter einem Substantiv eine Substanz anzunehmen, unter "Bewusstsein," "conscience" allmählich ein Ding zu verstehen; und wenn man sich gewöhnt hat, metaphorisch Lokalbeziehungen zuverwenden, wie "Unterbewusstsein," so bildet sich mit der Zeit wirklich eine Vorstellung aus, in der die Metapher vergessen ist und mit der man leicht manipuliert wie mit einer realen. Dann ist die Mythologie fertig.)[28]

Breuer's emphatic rejection of the substitution of abstract entities for persons as agents did not deter Freud from building an elaborate psychoanalytic mythology precisely on that *masquerade*. After his minimal collaboration with Freud, Breuer quickly dissociated himself from the psychoanalytic movement. I emphasize "minimal" because out of thirteen chapters in *Studies on Hysteria,* only one was coauthored. The other twelve are identified as either Breuer's or Freud's and are associated only by being bound together in a single volume. Clearly, Breuer wanted to play no part in Freud's pseudomedical adventure, built on an elaborate vocabulary of literalized metaphors.

V

During the half century between the 1880s, when Freud was a young physician, and the 1930s, when his work was finished, the medical-psychiatric scene became radically transformed. Psychogenic illnesses had become just another province in a vast pharmacratic empire.

In 1933, Karin (Costelloe) Stephen (1889–1953)—wife of Adrian Stephen, sister-in-law of Virginia (Stephen) Woolf—published a short book, titled *The Wish to Fall Ill,* in effect acknowledging that mental illnesses are counterfeit diseases. A more accurate title for her book would have been *The Wish to Be Excused and Pampered as If One Were Sick.* Stephen begins by emphasizing the differences between illnesses and nonillnesses:

In the history of medicine certain kinds of illness . . . have been peculiarly baffling. I mean the sort of symptoms which are often popularly spoken of as "hysterical" or "neurotic" or "mental." When there is something organically wrong with the body, when it has been injured or infected, medicine is at home. But in this other kind of illness, the doctor cannot find anything physical to account for the disturbance. In modern medicine the term *psychogenic* is used to cover this whole class of abnormalities whose origin appears to be *mental,* as contrasted with the more familiar *organic* illnesses in which the cause is *physical.*[29]

The difference between Stephen's rhetoric and Freud's is striking. Stephen accepts, as a fait accompli, the transformation of the *act of faking illness* into a *disease caused by the mind:* "Psychogenic illnesses presented a stumbling-block, so much so, indeed, that actually the word 'neurotic' degenerated into a term of abuse. It would almost seem as if doctors, *unable to deal with such patients,* had tried to comfort themselves by supposing that it was the patient's fault that he did not get well."[30]

Actually, many doctors were perfectly able to deal with such patients, by choosing to not deal with them. Under ordinary circumstances the relationship between doctors and patients is voluntary, similar to the relationship between salespersons and customers. They are free to choose to not have a relationship. Stephen knows this fact, and, precisely at this point, her common sense emerges from behind the screen of psychoanalytic jargon that pervades the rest of her book: "The doctor who says his neurotic patient is *being ill on purpose* is very near the truth."[31]

Stephen has a clear grasp of the existential function and meaning of mental illness as "the wish to be ill": "Of all the possibilities which they recognize as being open to them, their illness appears to them to be the least evil—*it has been created with extraordinary skill* to protect them from an even more terrible situation which seems to them to be the only alternative. It enables them to carry on somehow."[32]

These extracts from Stephen's book appear in the first five pages. Having unburdened herself of the truth, she lets her writing lapse into the base rhetoric of psychoanalytic jargon. After telling us about "personalities" that fragment and "dissociate," she begins her guided tour through the Alice in

Wonderland world of the hysteric: "A case occurred in which a wife, though she had the normal use of her eyesight for every other purpose, was unable to see her husband at all."[33] But there was no such case. There was only a woman, defined as a "patient," who offered this absurd account of her behavior, and a psychoanalyst, Karin Stephen, who seemingly accepted it on face value. I say "seemingly" because she concludes that "psychogenic illness" is ordinary behavior and therefore a nonillness: *Psychogenic illness is a piece of behavior as purposive as putting a hand up to ward off a blow.*[34]

Nevertheless, as a faithful member of the cult of psychoanalysis, Stephen rejected her commonsense perceptions and accepted the idea that counterfeit illness is also illness. It is an absurd—albeit in many ways convenient—way of interpreting and (mis)understanding human behavior.

VI

With its roots in psychiatry and the medicalization of unwanted behavior, it was easier to see through this piece of intellectual-moral mischief before Freud succeeded in merchandising it. In 1880, Jane Grey Swisshelm (1815–1884)—a now-forgotten abolitionist, feminist, and newspaperwoman—observed, "The diagnosis of drunkenness was that it was a disease for which the patient was in no way responsible, that it was created by existing saloons, and non-existing bright hearths, smiling wives, pretty caps and aprons. The cure was the patent nostrum of pledge-signing, a lying-made-easy invention, which like calomel, seldom had any permanent effect on the disease for which it was given, and never failed to produce another and a worse. Here the care created an epidemic of forgery, falsehood and perjury."[35]

Although the idea of removing responsibility from the actor by viewing his disapproved action as disease predates the invention of psychoanalysis, after Freud adopted this false doctrine as the basis of his "science," it became popular to blame him for it. Viennese journalist Karl Kraus noted that Freud was a quack almost as soon as Freud came to the attention of the Viennese public. In 1918, H. L. Mencken mocked his invention of the "unconscious deed" or "act-without-actor": "One of the laudable by-products of the Freudian quackery is the discovery that lying, in most cases, is involuntary and inevitable—that the liar can no more avoid it than he can avoid blinking his eyes when a light flashes or jumping when a bomb goes off behind him."[36]

Karl Jaspers (1883–1969)—better known as an existential philosopher than a psychiatrist, which is what he was until his forties—saw psychiatry clearly and fled the field. In his psychiatric magnum opus, *General Psycho-pathology*, first published in 1913, he wrote, "The behavior of neurotics and psychotics, criminals and eccentrics has been understood as a form of self-deception, a surrender to a fictitious existence."[37] Jaspers understood that, contrary to contemporary American psychiatric-sentimental rhetoric, mental patients do not "suffer" from an "illness"; on the contrary, they bask in the enjoyment of a special kind of self-indulgence:

> Gérard de Nerval [nom de plume of the French poet, essayist, and cel-ebrated suicide Gérard Labrunie (1808–1855)] began his description of his illness as follows: "I shall try to record the impression of a long illness that took place in the mysterious recesses of my mind. I do not know why I use the expression 'illness' because, as far as I am concerned, I never felt better in my life. Sometimes I took my powers and abilities as twice as great. I seemed to know and understand everything and my imagination gave me an immense delight."[38]

Under the heading "The Determination to Fall Ill," Jaspers wrote, "Patients want sympathy, want to create a sensation or evade some obligation, want to get a pension or enjoy certain fantasy pleasures. Determination and surren-der of this sort play a great part in neurotic illnesses as well as in the develop-ment of pseudologia phantastica (self-credited, fantastic lying)."[39]

The medicalization of malingering is the fatal genetic defect that dooms all theories and treatments of "mental diseases."

VII

Although medicalization encompasses more than psychiatry, we must be clear about one thing: *psychiatry is medicalization, through and through.* Whatever aspect of psychiatry psychiatrists claim is not medicalization is not medicalization only if it deals with proven disease, in which case it belongs to neurology, neuropathology, neurochemistry, neuropharmacology, or neurosurgery, not psychiatry.

Psychoanalysis is medicalization squared. It is important, in this connection, not to be fooled by lay analysis, clinical psychology, or social work. These and other nonmedical mental health and counseling "professions" are medicalizations cubed: as if to compensate for their lack of medical knowledge and medical privileges, nonmedical mental health "professionals" are even more deeply committed than psychiatrists to their claim of special expertise in the diagnosis and treatment of mental illnesses.[40]

Actually, by the time Sigmund Freud appeared on the historical stage, medicalization was in full swing: the birth of psychoanalysis is at once a manifestation of the increasing popularity of this trend at the end of the nineteenth century and a cause of its explosive growth during the twentieth century. In 1901 Freud published one of his favorite works, revealingly titled *The Psychopathology of Everyday Life*. The gist of Freud's thesis was that the symptoms of mental illnesses are the "products" of the same "mental processes" that are responsible for the thoughts and actions of normal persons. In other words, Freud rediscovered that "there is method in madness," or, as he preferred to put it, that sane and insane behaviors are subject to the same "psychological laws."

To create his special brand of pseudoscience, Freud titled his book *The Psychopathology of Everyday Life*. He could just as well have titled it *The Normality of Everyday Psychopathological Life*. However, there would have been neither fame nor fortune to follow. Instead, he fanned the flames of medicalization and transformed a smoldering fire into an all-consuming conflagration. At the same time, because he knew better, Freud's attitude toward medicalization was ambivalent and opportunistic. Most of the time, he was an enthusiastic medicalizer: "The neuroses are a particular kind of illness and analysis is a particular method of treating them, a specialized branch of medicine." He also wrote, "[The neuroses] are severe, constitutionally fixed illnesses, which rarely restrict themselves to only a few attacks but persist as a rule over long periods or throughout life." He also stated, "Psychoanalysis is really a method of treatment like others."[41] At other times, when it suited his purpose, Freud resisted the medicalization of psychoanalysis: "I have assumed, that is to say, that psychoanalysis is not a specialized branch of medicine. I cannot see how it is possible to dispute this." He continued: "In his medical school a doctor receives a training which is more or less the opposite of what he would need as a preparation for psychoanalysis." Finally, "We [analysts] serve the patient . . . as a teacher and educator."[42]

The honest psychoanalyst helps his patient come to terms with his secrets by promising to keep *secret* the information imparted to him in analysis, and keeping his promise. The psychoanalytic situation is modeled on the priest helping the penitent by promising to keep *secret* the information imparted to him in the confessional, and honoring the promise. The ethics of psychoanalysis is thus antithetical to the ethics of natural science: one values privacy, the other openness. Freud, however, wanted to eat his cake and have it too. With one hand, he unraveled—exposing the "method in madness" and demystifying mental illness. With the other hand, he raveled—legitimating fake illness as real illness, mystifying malingering as malady.

The debate about whether psychoanalysis (or any other form of psychotherapy) is a medical procedure is about law, not science. In the modern world, a procedure defined as medical treatment is, ipso facto, the property of the medical profession and hence of the state. The state prohibits the practice of medicine by persons not trained and licensed in medicine and punishes persons who violate this prohibition. By the same token, persons who are medically trained and licensed gain a monopoly for providing the particular service. The same struggle for power ensues when psychologists or other mental health workers seek to enlarge their professional privileges by, for example, aspiring to have the "right" to prescribe psychiatric incarceration or psychiatric drugs.

2 Doctoring

Doctor, v., to alter, falsify . . . to alter deceptively (accused of *doctoring* the election returns) (a *doctored* photo).

—Webster's Third New International Dictionary

By the time Freud came of age, the humoral concept of disease was an anachronism. The prescientific Galenic physician had been credited with therapeutic powers he did not possess, for curing diseases he could not objectively identify. In contrast, the modern scientific physician, basing his work on the methods of the natural sciences, made few, if any, therapeutic claims. During the nineteenth century, most such claims rightly carried the odor of charlatanry.

The scientific concept of disease is materialistic. Disease is an abnormal condition of the body, impairing its function. It was defined and detected by empirical study and by understanding the anatomy and physiology of the human body. The scientific physician's primary task was to objectively identify diseases, that is, make accurate clinical diagnoses, confirmed by postmortem diagnoses. By this definition, *mental disease* was, and remains, an oxymoron.

In 1881, Sigmund Freud finished his medical studies and was faced with the challenge of becoming an independent adult: moving out of the parental home, supporting himself, marrying and having a family of his own. In those days, the economic prospects of a young doctor in Vienna were poor, the opposite of what they are in the United States today.

In Austria-Hungary—and, after World War I, in Austria and Hungary—any young man or woman who graduated from an appropriate secondary school (gymnasium) had the right to enroll for a university degree. As a result, many more persons trained in medicine, and also in law, than had opportunities to earn a living practicing those professions. If the young doctor came from a family of modest means, as Freud did, his choices were limited. One of his options was to work his way up the ladder in academic medicine; another was to emigrate to the United States; a third was to settle for professionally demeaning employment (for example, as a "spa doctor" in a fashionable resort or as a mad-doctor in a provincial city, a job Chekhov portrays in *Ward No. 6*). A fourth choice, often taken, was to abandon medicine as a career and earn a living as, say, a businessman or writer.

Freud tried to pursue an academic career, but his poor performance in Ernst Brücke's laboratory put a finish to it. For more than four years, he drifted from one dead-end job to another. In 1885, Freud was twenty-nine years old, still living in the parental home, without sufficient income to support himself, uncomfortable in the role of practicing physician, full of ambition but unsure of how to satisfy his craving for prestige and power. He decided to become a disciple of the famous Parisian neurologist-neuropathologist Jean-Martin Charcot.

People believe that we fall in love because we are smitten by the admirable attributes—aesthetic, erotic, ethical, intellectual—of a particular person, profession, or "cause." More often it is the other way around. We fall in love because of our own need to love, to be bound closely to another person, vocation, or belief system. It was in this state of mind, it seems to me, that Freud decided to go to Paris, fall in love with Charcot, become certified as his "pupil," and engage in the practice of diagnosing and treating "nervous diseases"; or, put more precisely, *to become a specialist in the counterfeit diseases that Charcot had authenticated as real diseases, usually called "hysteria."*

Despite his important position and immense prestige, Charcot's deceptions did not go unnoticed. For example, Ernest-Charles Lasègue (1809–1883), a general physician and student of malingering, characterized hysteria as "the wastepaper basket of medicine where one throws otherwise unemployed symptoms." Lasègue died two years before Freud decided that the future of psychiatry lay in studying this nondisease. Even more sharply, neurologist Georges Gilles de la Tourette (1857–1904)—famous for his description of *"maladie des tics,"* now called "Tourette's syndrome"—declared, "You [Charcot] cultivate hysteria at the Salpêtrière, you don't cure it."[1]

"The most striking feature of the treatments employed [at the Salpêtrière]," observes historian Jan Goldstein in *Console and Classify,* a well-researched but uncritical history of nineteenth-century French psychiatry, "is their theatricality: Scenes and spectacles are staged. . . . These treatments are, to use a phrase of the period, 'pious frauds,' deceptions to take advantage of the gullibility of an individual for his own benefit."[2] Charcot's "pious frauds" at the Salpêtrière were the greatest show in Paris.

Skeptical physicians long ago recognized that there is no mystery about hysteria. It is not a disease and is not the name or diagnosis of a disease; instead, it is a collusive deception between a person playing disabled patient and a psychiatrist playing doctor diagnosing disease. This type of collusive medical deception is more common today than ever. Exposures of Charcot's deceptions did not diminish his iconic medical status. Similarly, none of the evidence that hysteria is a pious fraud has diminished the sacrosanct medicolegal status of psychiatry and its sacred symbol, "mental illness." Émile Zola aptly compared Charcot's cures with the cures at Lourdes and concluded that both were expressions of the human "hankering after the lie that forms the foundation of all religion."[3]

Freud traveled to Paris to be anointed by Charcot as an expert in hysteria. After his return to Vienna, he established himself as a physician specializing in nondiseases defined as diseases, following a path pioneered by the great Viennese charlatan Franz Anton Mesmer.

I

Who was this man, Charcot, with whom Freud fell in love and whose deceits he imitated and implemented with such enormous success? In 1885, when Freud met him, Charcot was sixty years old, a professor of neurology at the University of Paris, the most famous physician in France, the admired and feared "Caesar" of the Salpêtrière.

Correlating the signs and symptoms of patients suffering from various diseases with the pathoanatomical lesions found in their dead bodies, Charcot became one of the great scientific "clinicians" of his age. He observed, discovered/identified, and diagnosed/named several discrete disease entities. In 1852, when he was twenty-seven years old, he demonstrated, for the first time—by means of a test for uric acid—the objective differences between gout and so-called chronic arthritis (rheumatoid arthritis and osteoarthritis).[4]

Charcot was also a pioneer in the use of thermometry in medicine, emphasizing the superiority of rectal over axillary measurements. He was the first to describe intermittent claudication owing to arteriosclerosis, now usually called "peripheral artery disease," and made major contributions to the understanding of cerebral hemorrhage and Graves' disease (goiter, hyperthyroidism). There remains to be mentioned Charcot's most important work, on which his well-deserved fame rests: the identification of a score of diseases of the nervous system, including amyotrophic lateral sclerosis, multiple sclerosis, tabetic arthropathies, and "movement disorders," such as epilepsy and chorea. Only after these achievements did Charcot turn to the study of hysteria.

Before we consider the problem of hysteria-as-disease, we must keep in mind that, just as laypersons distinguish between voluntary actions and involuntary movements, so anatomists and physiologists distinguish between the voluntary nervous system and the involuntary nervous system. The concepts of voluntary-involuntary are indispensable for the formation of moral judgments and the administration of the law, as well as for the distinction between malingering as voluntary action and disease as involuntary happening.

Charcot solved the riddle of numerous afflictions by viewing the patients' abnormal behaviors—say, those actions owing to tabes dorsalis (a form of neurosyphilis)—as *involuntary,* attributable to lesions of the nervous system. This assumption proved richly rewarding. One can hardly blame him for assuming that the behaviors of persons "diagnosed" as hysterics were also *involuntary,* attributable to lesions of the nervous system. However, one can blame him for ignoring, indeed rejecting, the evidence that established, beyond the shadow of doubt, that hysterical symptoms were the *willed, voluntary actions* of the so-called patients.

By using the microscope to study the histology of the brains and spinal cords of cadavers, Charcot was able to see lesions of the central nervous system. Later, he turned to photography to similarly visualize and objectify what he took to be the lesions of "hysteria." But the photographic images of persons in various poses are in no way comparable to microscopic images of abnormal central nervous system tissues.

A brief digression about the history of photography and its use in medicine is in order here. In 1833, when Charcot was eight years old, Louis Daguerre (1789–1851) perfected an early method of photography named after him, the "daguerreotype." French neurologist and neurophysiologist Guillaume Duchenne (1806–1875), best known for identifying Duchenne muscular dystrophy (DMD, also known as muscular dystrophy, Duchenne type, a slowly fatal genetic disorder), pioneered in making photographic records of the clinical manifestations of neurological abnormalities. Charcot was Duchenne's pupil.

In 1862, at the age of thirty-seven, Charcot became the director of the Salpêtrière and created the greatest neurological clinic of the nineteenth century. Seeking to record the visible manifestations of neurological disorders in the movements of the body, he employed Desiré Magloire Bourneville (1840–1909) and Paul Régnard (1850–1927)—both physician pioneers in medical photography—to create a unique photographic chronicle of the patients at the Salpêtrière, mainly individuals diagnosed as hysterics whose performances were the most dramatic and photogenic. It became the legendary *Iconographie photographique de la Salpêtrière, Service de M. Charcot.*[5]

Qua neuropathologist studying hysteria, Charcot was like the proverbial workman whose only tool is a hammer and who therefore treats everything like a nail that needs hammering: he saw abnormal movements and treated them *as the symptoms of neurological disease (neuropathology)*. Freud, neuropathologist-turned-psychoanalyst, was like the crooked art collector who knowingly buys a forged masterpiece authenticated by experts as an original and resells it at a handsome profit: he saw abnormal behaviors and treated them *as if they were the symptoms of mental diseases (psychopathology)*.

II

Much has been written about Charcot, and I shall briefly review what various observers have discovered and concluded. I begin with Freud's impressions, which were the feelings of a love-struck young person divinizing his beloved. On November 24, 1885, barely a month after first laying eyes on Charcot, Freud writes to Martha Bernays, his future wife:

I think I am changing a great deal. I will tell you in detail what is affect-
ing me. Charcot, who is one of the greatest of physicians and a man whose
common sense is touched by genius, is simply uprooting my aims and opin-
ions. I sometimes come out of his lectures as though I were coming out
of Notre Dame, with a new idea of perfection. But he exhausts me; when
I come away from him I no longer have any desire to work at my own silly
things; it is three whole days since I have done any work, and I have no
feelings of guilt. My brain is sated, as if I had spent an evening at the theater. . . . [N]o one else has ever affected me in the same way.[6]

It is a remarkable letter to write to one's betrothed: "No one else has ever
affected me in the same way." Assuredly not Martha. Freud writes as if,
after listening to Charcot, he had come away from an overwhelming erotic-
existential experience, "exhausted," "sated." It is the sort of thing a man
might write after a memorable night of lovemaking or perhaps after listening to an hours-long speech by a great demagogue.

People abhor being baffled by the dangers that face them, which is why
they prefer false explanations to none and why we may fairly assert that people
have always "known" what causes diseases: demons, witches, the breaking of
taboo, the evil eye, wells poisoned by Jews, and, most enduringly, humoral
imbalances, as taught by Hippocrates and Galen. Bizarre, unpredictable
behaviors also baffle people and make them feel endangered. Attributing
such conduct to mental illnesses comforts them. It is for this reason that
people now "know" what causes mental diseases—bad brains, bad genes,
bad chemicals, bad societies, bad parents. The idea that there are no mental
diseases discomforts people and is therefore rejected.

Although Freud liked to claim that he had disturbed the sleep of mankind, the opposite is the case: he provided people with the comforts of a false
explanation. This falseness has been and is the source of the considerable
popularity of so-called Freudian ideas. In an early essay, titled "Hysteria"
(1888), Freud writes:

A proper assessment and a better understanding of the disease [hysteria]
only began with the works of Charcot and of the school of the Salpêtrière
inspired by him. Up to that time hysteria had been the *bête noire* of

medicine. The poor hysterics, who in earlier centuries had been burnt or exorcized, were only subjected, in recent, enlightened times, to the curse of the ridicule; their states were deemed unworthy of clinical observation, being simulation and exaggerations. Hysteria is a neurosis in the strict sense of the word—that is to say, not only have no perceptible changes in the nervous system been found in this illness, but it is not to be expected that any refinement of anatomical techniques would reveal any such changes. *Hysteria is based wholly and entirely on physiological modifications of the nervous system.*[7]

Freud had not a scintilla of evidence for this assertion, which, however, was necessary for classifying hysteria as a disease. Then, as now, when psychiatrists did not understand some aspect of human behavior, they glibly attributed it to "heredity." Freud did the same: "Hysteria must be regarded as a *status,* a nervous diathesis, which produces outbreaks from time to time. The aetiology of the *status hystericus* is to be looked for entirely in heredity."[8]

Freud insisted that neurosis is a disease, yet condemned the neurotic as a morally impaired person: "In a number of cases, to be sure, the hysteria is merely a symptom of a deep-going degeneracy of the nervous system which is manifested in permanent moral perversion." Accordingly, he endorsed coercion rationalized as cure: "The methods of earlier generations of physicians (who treated hysterical manifestations in young people as naughtiness and weakness of will and threatened them with punishment) were not bad ones, though they were hardly based on correct views."[9]

III

In 1893, when Charcot died, Freud wrote his obituary in the prestigious *Wiener Medizinische Wochenschrift.* He described the Master as follows:

He was not a reflective man, not a thinker: he had the nature of an artist—he was, as he himself said, a *"visuel,"* a man who sees. . . . The pupil who spent many hours with him going round the wards of the Salpêtrière—that museum of clinical facts, the names and peculiar characteristics of which were for the most part derived from him—would be reminded of Cuvier,

whose statue, standing in front of the *Jardin des Plantes,* shows that great
comprehender and describer of the animal world surrounded by a multi-
tude of animal forms; or else he would recall the myth of Adam, who, when
God brought the creatures of Paradise before him to be distinguished and
named may have experienced to the fullest degree that intellectual enjoyment which Charcot praised so highly.[10]

Here, Freud compares Charcot with God and mental patients with plants
or animals, objects to be named and controlled. In a similar vein, in his
"Preface and Footnotes to the Translation of Charcot's Tuesday Lectures"
(1892), Freud writes, "These lectures present so accurate a picture of Charcot's manner of speaking and thinking that, for anyone who has once sat
among his audience, the memory of the Master's [*sic*] voice and looks comes
alive once more and the precious hours return in which the magic of a great
personality bound his hearers irrevocably to the interests and problems of
neuropathology."[11] Since hysteria is a "disease" without a neuropathological
basis, Charcot's lectures on this subject had nothing to do with neuropathology, and Freud knew it. Nevertheless, he continued to characterize Charcot
with the naïveté of a starstruck teenager.

In 1893, Freud published another paper on hysteria, titled "Some Points
for a Comparative Study of Organic and Hysterical Motor Paralyses." He
states, "Hysteria has fairly often been credited with a faculty for *simulating*
the most various organic nervous disorders. . . . I, on the contrary, assert
that the lesion in hysterical paralyses must be completely independent of the
anatomy of the nervous system, since *in its paralyses and other manifestations
hysteria behaves as though anatomy did not exist or as though it had no knowledge of it.*" These writings are the earliest examples of what became Freud's
characteristically deceptive rhetoric, treating persons as objects, the vehicles
and victims of mental diseases, and psychiatric-psychoanalytic abstractions as
personalized agents with the power to *counterfeit* organic nervous disorders.
Freud then compounds the deception by asserting another falsehood: "For
this purpose [to distinguish hysterical from organic paralyses] [Charcot]
made use of hysterical patients whom he got into a state of somnambulism by
hypnotizing them. He succeeded in proving, by an unbroken chain of argument, that these paralyses were the result of ideas which had dominated the

patient's brain at moments of a special disposition. In this way, the mechanism of a hysterical phenomenon was explained for the first time."[12]

According to Georges Guillain, who spent many years at the Salpêtrière,
Charcot did not hypnotize any of the patients at the Salpêtrière. After the
sentences quoted above, Freud concludes: "This incomparably fine piece of
clinical research was afterward taken up by his own pupil, Pierre Janet, as
well as by Breuer and others, who developed from it a theory of neurosis
which coincided with the medieval view—when once they had replaced the
'demon' of clerical phantasy by a psychological formula."[13]

IV

Georges Charles Guillain (1876–1961) and his colleague Jean Alexander
Barré (1880–1967) are memorialized in neurology by the eponymous Guil-
lain-Barré syndrome, an often reversible polyneuropathy. Guillain deserves
to be remembered also for his definitive biography, *J.-M. Charcot, 1823–1893:
His Life—His Work,* an indispensable source for understanding Charcot's
work and the origin of modern psychopathology.

J.-M. Charcot consists of sixteen chapters and an epilogue, with only one
chapter devoted to "hysteria and the neuroses." In contrast to Freud, who
admired Charcot for his theatrical case presentations, Guillain lamented his
exhibitionism. So also did Pierre Janet (1859–1947) and neurologist Pierre
Marie (1853–1940), who writes, "For Charcot . . . the magisterial weekly
lecture in the amphitheatre was the grand event in life, the one that transcended all else, which was worked on during the week, which was meticulously rehearsed the morning before in the hospital, and which after the
giving of the lecture continued to be discussed late into the evening."[14]

Guillain's criticism of the Master is restrained, and is the more powerful
for it: "Without doubt some of these patients [at the Salpêtrière] were agile
comedians and excellent imitators. Moreover, the assistants and interns of
Charcot made the mistake of having them repeat their spectacular crises in
front of physicians and medical students."[15] Every player in this drama was an
actor, in the dual sense of the term. Everyone was a performer in a carefully
choreographed play, admired and applauded by *tout Paris.* At the same time,
Guillain emphasizes:

Charcot had recognized the role played by emotion, imagination, suggestion, fabrication, and prevarication in all hysteric phenomena. . . . Charcot, for example, was very much aware of the malingering found among some hysterics. In one of his lectures he said: "This brings me to say a few words about malingering. It is found in every phase of hysteria and one is surprised at times to admire the ruse, the sagacity, and the unyielding tenacity that especially the women, who are under the influence of a severe neurosis, display in order to deceive, especially when the victim of the deceit happens to be a physician."[16]

Charcot's penchant for self-dramatization and showmanship made him an easy mark for such deceptions. He was aware of this weakness but apparently made little effort to resist it. In an address at the Salpêtrière, he spoke "about the difficulties that the clinician encounters in the study of the neuroses . . . [which have] to do with simulation, not that sort of imitation of one disease by another of which we just spoke, but rather intentional malingering, in which the patient voluntarily exaggerates real symptoms or even creates in every detail an imaginary symptomatology. Indeed, everyone is aware of the human need to lie . . . and this is particularly true in hysteria."[17] In short, Charcot was not an innocent victim of scheming hysterics; he was a knowing conspirator in one of the greatest medical hoaxes of the modern age.

Guillain was not about to challenge the "myth of mental illness" in *statu nascendi* but powerful even as an infant. Ignoring his own evidence, he continues with a description of Charcot's method of treating the disease: "I remind you, gentlemen, that there are two parts in the treatment of hysteria . . . the psychic element . . . and the physical element. . . . It is also evident that static electricity deserves a place in this regimen of physical therapy."[18]

Unquestionably, Charcot was one of the giants of late-nineteenth-century French medicine and neurology. This status may be why psychiatrists and psychiatric historians have failed to see that he was *also a quack,* albeit a new kind of quack. The old quacks—such as Franz Mesmer and Mary Baker Eddy—duped people into believing that fake cures were real cures. The new quacks—such as Charcot and Freud—duped people into believing that fake diseases were real diseases.

The basis for this new quackery—the mutual lie, patient and doctor alike pretending to believe his own and (some of) his partner's prevarications—lay in the social structure of psychiatric practice, a structure that had been in place since the French Revolution and before. Charcot's contribution consisted in lending the weight of his persona and prestige to authenticating this mutual deception as not only medical diagnosis but also medical treatment. It is important to note here that one of Charcot's favorite therapeutic methods for hysteria was *psychiatric incarceration*: "The isolation of patients afflicted with hysteric psychoneuroses always preoccupied Charcot. . . . '[W]e must separate both children and adults from their fathers and their mothers whose influence, as experience has shown, is particularly pernicious.'"[19]

Despite Guillain's consistently hagiographic tone, in the penultimate chapter of his book, titled "Hypnotism," he acknowledges that Charcot betrayed his obligation to truth-telling: "Charcot obviously made a mistake in not checking his experiments. . . . [H]is chiefs of clinics, his interns, and other assistants prepared the patients, hypnotized them, and organized the experiments. Charcot personally never hypnotized a single patient, never checked the experiments and, as a result, was not aware of their inadequacies or of the reasons of their eventual errors."[20] Charcot's character traits cannot be excused as "mistakes." He wanted to be a medical showman and despot, and that's what he became. "I cannot ignore, however," Guillain continues,

> a question that has often come to my mind. Charcot has assistants of high scientific caliber, gifted with a penetrating and critical type of mind, who possessed high moral integrity. It seems to me impossible that some of them did not question the unlikelihood of certain contingencies. Why did they not put Charcot on their guard? The only explanation that I can think of, with all the reservation that it carries, is that they did not dare alert Charcot, fearing the violent reactions of the master, who was called the "Caesar" of the Salpêtrière.[21]

Near the end of his account, Guillain quotes the recollections of Georges Guinon (1859–1932), Charcot's last "private secretary" and later himself a noted neurologist. In 1925—that is, thirty-two years after the death of the Caesar of the Salpêtrière—Guinon wrote:

I have some very vivid recollections of a conversation that I had with Charcot a short time before his death. . . . He told me that his concept of hysteria had become decadent and his entire chapter on the pathology of the nervous system must be revised. . . . Charcot had foreseen the need of dismembering his theory on hysteria and was preparing himself to dynamite the edifice to which he had personally contributed so much in building. Is it not interesting that perhaps I am the only one today to be aware of this fact?[22]

Guillain follows the chapter "Hysteria and the Neuroses" with a chapter titled "Babinski's Theories of Hysteria." Joseph Babinski (1857–1932)—another in the long line of distinguished late-nineteenth- and early-twentieth-century French neurologists—discovered the Babinski sign, also called the plantar reflex, a simple but important indication of disease or injury to the central nervous system. What Babinski did with hysteria is what psychiatrists do whenever they are embarrassed about writing about a nondisease as if it were a disease—he changed its name: "We can give to these disturbances the name 'pithiatic.' [Amenable to suggestion] . . . The adjective 'pithiatic' would substitute for 'hysteric.'"[23]

For the psychiatrist, the important thing in all this hocus-pocus is to define malingering as disease and keep legal-political control over the subject as mental patient. "My observation of the vast numbers of hysterics," concluded Babinski, " . . . led me to the conviction, *which is also shared by all neurologists,* that many of these subjects are sincere and cannot be considered as malingerers."[24] Doctors have no way of knowing which of their patients is sincere.

V

No review of hysteria-as-lying by patient and physician alike would be complete without reference to one of the great international best-sellers of the twentieth century, *The Story of San Michele* (1929), by Swedish physician-writer Axel Munthe (1857–1949). I read this book as a teenager growing up in Budapest, and it made a lasting impression on me. Years later, I reread it in English, and read it once more in preparation for writing this book.

Munthe, multilingual scion of a noble Swedish family, studied medicine in Uppsala, Montpellier, and Paris, where he was a student of Charcot. He married an aristocratic English woman, wrote *The Story of San Michele* in English, was a lover of art, and lived in Italy during much of his life. In 1887, he moved to Capri and purchased the Villa San Michele, hence the title of his largely autobiographical book. In the chapter titled "Doctors," Munthe describes Charcot with these words:

> He never admitted a mistake and woe to the man who ever dared to hint at his being in the wrong. . . . Charcot was the most celebrated doctor of his time. . . . His voice was imperative, hard, often sarcastic. The grip of his small, flabby hand was unpleasant. He had few friends among his colleagues. . . . He was indifferent to the suffering of his patients, he took little interest in them from the day of establishing the diagnosis until the day of the post-mortem examination. . . . [The] stage performances of the Salpêtrière before the public of tout Paris were nothing but an absurd farce, a hopeless muddle of truth and cheating.[25]

These lines were written some forty years after Munthe witnessed Charcot's performances that so captivated Freud. "I had already then," Munthe explains, "grave doubts as to the correctness of Charcot's theories, accepted without opposition by his blindfolded pupils and the public by means of what can only be explained as a sort of suggestion *en masse*."[26]

Munthe realized that the uneducated young women Charcot used as circus performers were, *de facto* or *de lege*, prisoners of the Salpêtrière, and this awareness upset him greatly: "One Sunday as I was leaving the hospital, I came upon a pair of old peasants sitting under the plane trees in the inner court." He learns that the visitors want to see their twenty-year-old daughter, Geneviève, who had come to the Salpêtrière two years earlier to work as a kitchen maid. Munthe realizes that Geneviève is Charcot's star performer, his most spectacular "hysteric," and undertakes to "save" her. He takes Geneviève home and tries to engineer her escape—an early example of a failed attempt to "deinstitutionalize" mental patients who have made the asylum their home. Geneviève betrays Munthe. The next day, when he shows up at the Salpêtrière, he is told Charcot wishes to speak to him:

Speaking very slowly, his deep voice trembling with rage, he said I had tried to allure to my house an inmate of his hospital, a young girl, a deséquilibrée, half unconscious of her acts. . . . I answered angrily that it was he and his followers and not I who had brought ruin to this girl who had entered the hospital as a strong and healthy peasant girl and would leave it as a lunatic if she remained there much longer. I had adopted the only course open to me to return her to her old parents. I had failed to rescue her and I was sorry I had failed. *"Assez, Monsieur!"* he shouted.[27]

Munthe is barred from entering the Salpêtrière again. So ends the chapter titled "Salpêtrière." The next chapter of *The Story of San Michele* is titled "Hypnotism," which begins as follows: "The famous platform performances in the amphitheatre of the Salpêtrière which brought on my disgrace, have since long been condemned by every serious student of hypnotic phenomena."[28] Alas, this statement is not true. Hypnosis is alive and well.[29] Munthe concludes: "The fact that the person cannot be hypnotized without his or her will, must not be overlooked. . . . Of course, all talk about an unwilling and unaware person being hypnotized at a distance is sheer nonsense. So also is Psycho-Analysis."[30]

VI

"Sheer nonsense" has always been at home in the business of consoling men and women for being human and offering to remove the burdens of that condition from their shoulders. Religion in its many incarnations, phrenology, mesmerism, hypnosis, psychoanalysis—all played this role. All the while, new players crowd the wings, eager to occupy center stage. Today, the new stars locate the mind in the brain and research "consciousness," neuroimaging brains that "light up," doctors "give" patients "drug therapy" as well as "talk therapy" and tell the public that both work by "changing the brain." A Mick Stevens cartoon in the January 29, 2007, issue of the *New Yorker* mocks this modern confusion. Captioned "Good shrink, bad shrink," it shows a patient lying on a couch placed between two psychiatrists sitting to each side. One shrink tells the patient, "Face your demons," while the other says, "Take a pill."

Unhappiness, desperation, disappointment, and suicide are part and parcel of the human condition. They are owing neither to possession by demons nor to diseases of the mind. Everyone knows it, but not everyone has the courage to believe it, much less to assert it. Meanwhile, the business of (mis)diagnosing people as suffering from mental illnesses and mistreating them with drugs, electricity, surgery, and conversation grows apace. And no cartoonist, no columnist, no mental health educator, no establishment psychiatrist or psychologist dares to mention the proverbial elephant in the room—coercion.

Today more than ever, psychiatry is a combination of pseudoneurology and the use of state-sponsored force, a sand castle of abstractions (consciousness, the unconscious, mental illness, chemical imbalance) masquerading as agents. The last prominent medical personage to recognize the ruinous presence of the elephant and tell the truth about psychiatry was Silas Weir Mitchell, founder of the American Neurological Association. In 1894, the American Medico-Psychological Association—now the American Psychiatric Association—invited Mitchell to present a special address at the fiftieth anniversary celebration of the group's first meeting. With misgivings, Mitchell agreed and delivered a scathing lecture, telling the assembled mad-doctors:

> You quietly submit to having hospitals called asylums; you are labeled as medical superintendents. . . . You should urge in every report the stupid folly of this. You . . . conduct a huge boarding house—what has been called a monastery of the mad. . . . I presume that you have, through habit, lost the sense of jail and jailor which troubles me when I walk behind one of you and he unlocks door after door. Do you think it is not felt by some of your patients. . . . *You have for too long maintained the fiction that there is some mysterious therapeutic influence to be found behind your walls and locked doors. We hold the reverse opinion. . . . Your hospitals are not our hospitals; your ways are not our ways.*[31]

More than ever, the ways of psychiatry are not the ways of (traditional) medicine, and more than ever the ways of medicine resemble the ways of psychiatry.

3 Inculpating

In the priest, as in the psychiatrist *[aliénist]*, there is always something
of the examining magistrate.

—Marcel Proust (1871–1922), quoted in *Console and*
Classify, by Jan Goldstein

Is psychiatry a science? Is psychoanalysis a science? Are they medical sciences? Are they medical practices? At present, in the United States, the proposition that psychiatric and psychoanalytic practices are instances of medical practices is an article of faith promoted and protected by the power of the (therapeutic) state.

The (physical) scientist studies nature. He explains *material* phenomena by reference to their causes, that is, the preexisting events that "determine" their present state. In Freud's day, this understanding is what was meant by "determinism," the opposite of which was dismissively called "belief in free will." This understanding is still the case among scientists who view belief in free will as similar to belief in superstitions. Freud was deeply committed to the claim that psychoanalysis is a natural science and hence requires the denial of free will. He adopted this position early in his career and never budged from it.

He was not alone. Psychology, like psychoanalysis, is a novel human invention and a new academic discipline. Both are fallouts of the Enlightenment, modernity, the age of science—and pseudoscience. While Freud was developing the "science of psychoanalysis" in Europe, William James (1842–1910) was developing the "science of psychology" in the United States. Trained as a physician, James began his career teaching physiology to medical students. Unlike Freud, James knew, deep in his heart, that psychology is not a science and could not be one. But, like Freud, he too wished it were a science. Freud went further than mere wishing: he created a mythical science and a web of "discoveries." James—a true religious believer—wished it into being. In 1892, in an essay revealingly titled "A Plea for Psychology as a Natural Science," James writes, "I wished, by treating Psychology *like* a natural science, to help her to become one."[1] It's like a child wishing that by treating his hobby horse like a pony, it will become one.

Such candor was not Freud's dish. In 1901, in *The Psychopathology of Everyday Life,* Freud frames his claim that psychoanalysis is a science as follows: "If the distinction between conscious and unconscious motivation is taken into account, our feeling of conviction informs us that conscious motivation does not extend to all our motor decisions. . . . [W]hat is thus left free by the one side receives its motivation from the other side, from the unconscious; and in this way determination in the psychical sphere is still carried out without any gap."[2] For the rest of his life, Freud worked and reworked this fatuous claim.

In *An Outline of Psychoanalysis* (1938), written at the end of his life, Freud dismisses philosophy and "the psychology of consciousness" and lavishes praise on his own creation, psychoanalysis: "Whereas the psychology of consciousness never went beyond the broken sequences which were obviously dependent on something else, the other view, which held that *the psychical is unconscious in itself, enables psychology to take its place as a natural science [Naturwissenschaft] like any other.* The processes with which it is concerned are in themselves just as knowable as those dealt with by the other sciences, by chemistry or physics, for example."[3] This statement is patently false. Chemists and physicists analyze material objects; psychoanalysts "analyze" the *meaning* of dreams and the (mis)conduct of persons.

Freud knew it, of course. So instead of saying that psychoanalysts analyze material objects, he says they analyze "some kind of energy": "We assume, as other natural sciences have led us to expect, that in mental life some kind of energy is at work. . . . [T]his hypothesis [about the "psychical apparatus"] has put us in a position to establish psychology on foundations similar to those of any other science, such, for instance, as physics."[4] Finally, in a brief essay written shortly before his death, Freud reiterates that "psychology, too, is a natural science [*Naturwissenschaft*]. What else can it be?"[5] The answer, especially in German, is painfully obvious: a *Geisteswissenschaft.*

Analogies and metaphors may be useful explanatory devices or misleading similes. In no case can an imagined or hypothesized entity be evidence of its existence as a real or physical entity. Wilhelm Reich (1897–1957), one of the giants in the early history of psychoanalysis, owes his fame largely to having carried Freud's baseless assumption about "mental energy" to its absurd and tragic conclusion: he believed and claimed that Freud's fictitious energy was real, "bioelectrical" energy, called it "orgone," and maintained that he could capture and concentrate it in a machine he invented and called the "orgone accumulator" and "orgone generator."[6]

I

Freud spent a good deal of effort to establish the scientific bona fides of psychoanalysis. In 1914, in his essay "On the History of the Psycho-analytic Movement," he characterizes his work as a scientific "discovery" and appraises his role in the history of science in terms that border on megalomania. Apropos of his 1896 lecture to the Vienna Society for Psychiatry and Neurology on "the sexual factors involved in the *causation of my patients' neuroses,*" he writes as if it were self-evident that neuroses are neuropathological diseases and that "sexual factors" (whatever that term might have meant) are their *causes.* Here Freud acts as if he had forgotten that, like Charcot, he had stated that hysteria is *not* a neuropathological illness. Offering no evidence that neuroses are diseases (in the then accepted sense of the term), his lecture is received with icy silence. That convinces Freud that he is a great scientific pioneer: "I understood that from now onwards I was one of those who 'have disturbed the sleep of the world,' as Hebbel says. . . . I was prepared to accept the fate that sometimes accompanies such discoveries." In the rest of the essay, he asserts and reasserts the medical-scientific character of psychoanalysis: "With this incomplete outline I have attempted to give some idea of the still incalculable wealth of connections which have come to light between medical psychoanalysis and other fields of science."[7]

Finally, in 1917, Freud famously compares himself with Copernicus and Darwin. Copernicus demonstrated that the earth is not the center of the universe, delivering the first "blow to human narcissism." Darwin demonstrated that man is an animal, the second such "blow," and Freud that "the ego is not master in its own house," the third "blow."[8]

Freud's self-image as a disturber of the sleep of the world and subverter of self-love is deliciously distorted and conceited. His invention, psychoanalysis, resting on abstract nouns replacing human actors, makes Freud one of modernity's greatest semantic anesthesiologists and boosters of narcissism. Can anyone today doubt that Freud elevated navel gazing to new heights or that psychoanalysis increased the sum total of narcissism in the world, especially for its practitioners and devotees?

By creating imaginary entities—"id," "ego," "superego"—Freud alienates us from the simple truth that mental illnesses are endogenic (self-caused) phenomena that belong in the same class as do other medicalized endogenic phenomena, such as malingering and murder, and differ radically from exogenic (externally caused) phenomena, such as malaria and melanoma. Promising to demystify mental illnesses, Freud deepens the mystery by attributing the "etiology" of the "illness" to the patient's "unconscious mind." The result is a split between *acts and agents,* creating, as Sartre aptly puts it, *lies without liars.*[9]

Freud's unexamined and never-to-be examined premise is that neuroses are diseases yet unlike other diseases: "In certain diseases—including the very neuroses of which we have made special study—things are different. . . . The ego feels uneasy; it comes up against limits to its power in its own house, the mind. Thoughts emerge suddenly without one's knowing where they come from, nor can one do anything to drive them away." If we replace "ego" with "person," the statement becomes simplistic. Freud precludes such interpretation by reifying the ego: "The ego says to itself: 'This is an illness, a foreign invasion,'" and congratulates himself for imparting meaning to "mental symptoms" that psychiatrists dismiss as meaningless:

> Psychiatry, it is true, denies that such things mean the intrusion into the mind of evil spirits from without; beyond this, however, it can only say with a shrug: "Degeneracy, hereditary disposition, constitutional inferiority." Psychoanalysis sets out to explain these uncanny disorders, until at length

it can speak thus to the ego: "Nothing has entered into you from without; a part of the activity of your own mind has been withdrawn from the command of your will. . . . The blame, I am bound do say, lies with yourself. You over-estimated your strength when you thought you could treat your sexual instincts as you liked and could utterly ignore their intentions. The result is that they have rebelled."[10]

Freudian "explanation" is an example of base rhetoric.[11] At the beginning of his medical career—before there was such a thing as psychoanalysis and its mendacious-metaphoric language—Freud was well aware of the differences between hard science and storytelling. In *Studies on Hysteria* (1893–1895), he writes:

I have not always been a psychotherapist. Like other neuropathologists, I was trained to employ local diagnoses and electro-prognosis, and it still strikes me as strange that the case histories I write should read like short stories and that, as one might say, they lack the serious stamp of science [*Wissenschaftlichkeit;* scientificness]. I must console myself with the reflection that the nature of the subject is evidently responsible for this, rather than any preference of my own.[12]

When Freud wrote these lines, the last thing he wanted to do was cut the umbilical cord that tied him to medicine and provided him with professional legitimacy and prestige. Using the passive voice, he disavows that he is the author of his "case histories": "I must console myself with the reflection that the nature of the subject is evidently responsible for this, rather than any preference of my own." Said in metaphor/jest, but meant literally/in earnest. What began as *façons de parler* became the building blocks of the pseudoscience of psychoanalysis.

Freud always knew that psychoanalysis was not real science. He protested but, in the back of his mind-conscience, he knew better. "It may be pointed out," he noted in his essay "The Claims of Psychoanalysis to Scientific Interest" (1913), "that the interpretations made by psychoanalysis are first and foremost translations from an alien method of expression into the one which is familiar to us."[13]

II

Whenever we quote Freud we must be aware that Freud wrote in German and we are quoting his translators. Few writers have been translated with as much care as Sigmund Freud. *The Standard Edition of the Complete Psychological Works of Sigmund Freud* was prepared under the general editorship of James Strachey, a former patient and a friend of Freud, brother of the famous Lytton Strachey. He was assisted by his wife, Alix Strachey, and by Alan Tyson, both prominent English psychoanalysts. The entire project was supervised and approved by Anna Freud. Yet, or rather because of it, the result is imperfect, as several critics have noted.

Like other nonnative speakers of English, I am acutely aware that there are many expressions in a language that are all but untranslatable into another language. Two of the most relevant examples of the absence of linguistic congruence between German and English pertain to two common terms, *mind* and *science*. There is no German equivalent for the English word *mind,* either as a noun or as a verb. Usually, it is translated as *Seele* (soul), or *Geist* (spirit). Mental illness is *Seelenkrankheit* or *Geisteskrankheit*.[14] In German, there is also no word for *science,* in the comprehensive sense in which English-speaking persons use the term. The *New Cassell's German Dictionary* renders *science* as *Wissenschaft* and *Wissenschaft* as "learning, knowledge, scholarship, science." In Latin, *scientia (ae)* means "knowledge" or "skill." These linguistic differences have acquired far-reaching implications with the growth of the hard sciences using mathematical or other specialized symbols as their languages and their differentiation from the moral or human sciences, anchored in ethics and philosophy and using ordinary language, albeit with extraordinary care and precision.

One of the most thoughtful commentaries on Freud-in-translation is *Freud and Man's Soul,* by Bruno Bettelheim (1903–1990), a Viennese lay analyst. According to Bettelheim, "The purpose of Freud's lifelong struggle was to help us understand ourselves, that we would no longer be propelled by forces unknown to us. . . . Introspection is what psychoanalysis is all about."[15] Alas, if only that were true. Introspection is, inter alia, what psychoanalysis *ought* to be about. But introspection is not a treatment, much less a science. Had psychoanalysis been essentially about introspection, Freud would have been a philosopher in the tradition of Socrates, a role he systematically rejected in favor of the role of natural scientist. Bettelheim explains:

> In the German culture within which Freud lived, and which permeated his work, there existed and still exists a definite and important division between two approaches to knowledge. Both disciplines are called *Wissenschaften* (sciences; literally *knowledge*), and they are accepted as equal in their approaches to their fields, although their methods have hardly anything in common. These two are the *Naturwissenschaften* (natural sciences) and, opposed to them in content and in methods, the *Geisteswissenschaften*. The term *Geisteswissenschaften* defies translation into English; its literal meaning is "sciences of the spirit," and the concept is one that is deeply rooted in German idealist philosophy.[16]

Although no term completely defies translation, *Geisteswissenschaft* is, indeed, challenging. In plural form, as *Geisteswissenschaften,* the term refers to the disciplines that used to be called the moral sciences or humanities and are now called the social sciences or behavioral sciences. The latter term is particularly misleading, as Jacques Barzun had pointed out, replacing it with the apt term *misbehavioral sciences.*[17]

German philosopher Wilhelm Windelband (1848–1915) described the differences between the terms *Naturwissenschaft* and *Geisteswissenschaft*—which gained currency only in the nineteenth century—as follows. The *Naturwissenschaften* (plural form), exemplified by the physics, characterized by extraspection and the use of the third-person pronoun, are concerned with objective phenomena and aim at the formulation of general laws, whereas the *Geisteswissenschaften,* exemplified by psychology, characterized by introspection and the use of the first-person pronoun, are concerned with unique personal behavior or past events, and aim at the understanding of particular occurrences and subjective phenomena. Windelband called the former "nomothetic," the latter "idiographic." Psychology and psychoanalysis are typical idiographic sciences. Not by coincidence, one of Windelband's major works was titled *On Free Will,* the concept against which Freud waged a lifelong battle. Freud never mentions Windelband, never uses the terms *nomothetic* and *idiographic,* and ignores the notions of individual liberty and responsibility, ideas rightly alien to the *Naturwissenschaften.*

In English-speaking countries, "hard scientists," professionals whose language is mathematics or other scientific symbols (as in chemistry), often do not regard "soft scientists," whose only language is *ordinary language,* as real scientists. Physicians are considered scientists because they use special physical-chemical methods for diagnosing and treating objectively identifiable diseases (of the body). If and when psychiatrists are considered scientists, it is because, allegedly, they too use special medical methods for diagnosing and treating brain diseases called "mental diseases." Bettelheim's conclusion is correct: "Psychoanalysis is plainly an idiographic science, utilizing unique historical occurrences to provide a view of man's development and behavior. . . . [H]e is working within the framework of *Geisteswissenschaften,* applying the methods appropriate to an idiographic science."[18] What else could psychoanalysis—based entirely on a private conversation between two persons—be?

III

In *New Introductory Lectures on Psychoanalysis* (1933), Freud reiterates his claim that psychoanalysis is a morally and politically neutral (natural) science:

> *"Weltanschauung"* is, I am afraid, a specifically German concept, the translation of which into a foreign language might well raise difficulties. . . . [A] *Weltanschauung* is an intellectual construction which solves all the problems of our existence uniformly on the basis of *one overriding hypothesis.* . . . If that is the nature of a *Weltanschauung,* the answer as regards psychoanalysis is made easy. As a specialized science, a branch of psychology—a depth-psychology or psychology of the unconscious—it is quite unfit to construct a *Weltanschauung* of its own; it must accept the scientific one. . . . [S]ince the *intellect and the mind are objects for scientific research in exactly the same way as any other non-human thing* . . . [psychoanalysis's] contribution to science lies precisely in having extended research to the mental field. . . . Of the three powers which may dispute the basic position of science, religion alone is to be taken seriously as an enemy.[19]

These ideas are painfully conventional and misguided. In Europe in 1933, religion was not the enemy of science; scientism qua psychology and scientific materialism was. When people like Copernicus and Newton studied nature, they regarded their work in essentially religious terms. They were studying God's handiwork: created by God, the universe worked according to certain rules or laws; discovering what those laws were was a way to discover and know more about God. This outlook protected them from the scientistic political megalomania that came to dominate Freud's world, and ours.

Freud was politically naive and temperamentally autocratic. He was oblivious to the fact that, in the modern world, ideas and practices officially considered scientific often have a profound influence on law and politics, whereas those concepts classified as religious do not, and that the politicization of science may be harmful to the liberty and well-being of certain individuals and groups just as formerly the politicization of religion had been. This point was obvious to many in 1933. Five years later, Freud and his family were among the victims of the pseudoscience whose nature he never grasped.

Blinded by his "cause," Freud failed to see that his claim that psychoanalysis is a natural science is a lie that will come back to haunt him and, perhaps more important, haunt his legacy. In *Introductory Lectures on Psychoanalysis* (1915–1917), Freud compares the analyst's task with the work of a detective: "And if you were a detective engaged in tracing a murder, would you expect to find that the murderer had left his photograph behind at the place of the crime, with his address attached? Or would you not have to be satisfied with comparatively slight and obscure traces of the person you were in search of?" Freud uses this analogy to explain why seemingly insignificant slips of the tongue are *clues*. To what? To a secret the speaker wishes to hide that is the *crucial link in a causal chain*: "If anyone makes a breach of this kind in the determinism of natural events at a single point, it means that he has thrown overboard the whole *Weltanschauung* of science."[20]

The analogy between disease and crime, analyst and detective, ensnares Freud in a simile of his own making: "When someone charged with an offense confesses his deed to the judge, the judge believes his confession; but if he denies it, the judge does not believe him. If it were otherwise, there would be no administration of justice." The judicial procedure Freud describes harks back to what we would call "inquisitorial justice." Adopting the format of a dialogue with an imaginary interlocutor, Freud makes his opponent conclude: "'Are you a judge, then? And is the person who has made a slip of the tongue brought up before you on a charge? So making a slip of the tongue is an offense, is it?'" Freud's response to this logical inference is to dismiss his interlocutor as self-deceived: "'You nourish the illusion of there being such a thing as psychical freedom, and you will not give it up. I am sorry to say I disagree with you categorically over this.'" Later, he reasserts: "'[If you believe in free will,] then you are making a big mistake. Once before I ventured to tell you that you nourish a deeply rooted faith in undetermined psychical events and in free will, but that this is quite unscientific and must yield to the demand of a determinism whose rule extends over mental life.'"[21] Obsessed with "psychic determinism," Freud ignores that we customarily explain events by attributing them to causes, and actions by attributing them to motives or reasons.

More than fifty years ago, Jean-Paul Sartre (1905–1980) recognized the conundrum Freud had created with his notion of "psychic determinism" and the fictitious mental entity "the unconscious" endowed with agency: "The profound contradiction in all psychoanalysis, is that it presents *at the same time* a bond of causality and a bond of understanding between the phenomena that it studies. These two types of relationships are incompatible. . . . [W]e do not reject the findings of psychoanalysis when they are obtained by the understanding. We limit ourselves to the denial that there is any value or intelligibility in its underlying theory of psychic causality." Elsewhere, Sartre states, "Thus psychoanalysis substitutes for the notion of bad faith the idea of a lie without a liar; it allows me to understand how it is possible for me to be lied to without lying to myself since it places me in the same relation to myself as the Other is in respect to me; it replaces the duality of the deceiver and the deceived, the essential condition of the lie, by that of the 'id' and the 'ego.'"[22]

Freud was a raconteur, not a scientist. Apropos of the similarities between the tales told by Freud and Conan Doyle, Adam Kirsch, the book editor of the *New York Sun*, writes:

The secluded study, the thoughtful silences, the brilliant deductive leaps, even the cocaine addiction—there is no mistaking the similarity between

Freud and Sherlock Holmes. Freud's case studies of the Wolfman and the Ratman share the suspense and glamour of Conan Doyle's tales of the Red-Headed League or the Speckled Band. Someone comes to Freud with a nightmare of six white wolves perched in a tree, or an obsessive fear of horses. The doctor, like the detective, is not deeply interested in legwork: Instead he sits in his study, listening quietly as the evidence forms a pattern in his mind, and then triumphantly names the culprit. Of course, in Freud's world the guilty party is always the victim himself, wearing the disguise of the unconscious—it is his own lusts and shames that have left him phobic or paranoid.[23]

IV

Freud saw himself as the "discoverer of a new science." Others see him as the leader of a cult.[24] Although he claimed that psychoanalysis was a treatment, he was not particularly interested in helping patients. Instead, he was interested in penetrating the "secrets" of artists and in exposing "fakes." When his friend and colleague Theodor Reik (1888–1969) compared him with Holmes, Freud said he would prefer to be compared with Giovanni Morelli, a nineteenth-century art scholar famous for his skill in "detecting fakes."[25]

Freud was too eager to see himself as a crime buster: "I must draw an analogy between the criminal and the hysteric," he writes in 1906. "In both we are concerned with a secret, with something hidden." This analogy is part of the larger theme of Freud's metaphors, masterfully explored in *The Tangled Bank* by Stanley Edgar Hyman (1919–1970), a now-forgotten literary critic. Yet even Hyman—keenly aware of Freud's metaphoric style—overlooked the most obvious and most important Freudian metaphor of all, namely, psychopathology: "In recognizing the hysteric to be genuinely ill rather than malingering," Hyman writes, "Charcot was the liberator."[26] Hyman fails to free himself of the incubus of malingering that has haunted psychiatry—and psychoanalysis perhaps even more—from its inception.

Hyman emphasizes Freud's fondness for comparing the method of psychoanalysis with the methods of detecting crimes and art forgeries. "We can see," he remarks, "Conan Doyle's hand in the titles Freud gives the dreams, so like Holmes cases: 'The Dream of Irma's Injection,' 'The Dream of the Botanical Monograph.'" In "The Moses of Michelangelo," Freud puts it thus: "It seems to me [Morelli's] method of inquiry is closely related to the technique of psychoanalysis. It, too, is accustomed to divine secret and concealed things from unconsidered or unnoticed details, from the rubbish-heap, as it were, of our observations."[27]

Freud acknowledges that his interest in other people's lives resembles the forensic pathologist's interest in the corpses of persons who die under suspicious circumstances. Artists who knew him were not pleased. Stefan Zweig, the author of an admiring minibiography of Freud, writes, "If Nietzsche philosophizes with a hammer, Freud philosophizes with a scalpel." Thomas Mann was more emphatic: "As an artist, I have to confess, however, that I am not at all satisfied with Freudian ideas; rather, I feel disquieted and reduced by them. The artist is being x-rayed by Freud's ideas to the point where it violates the secret of his creative art."[28]

As I noted earlier, comparing the analyst's efforts with the work of a detective is moral suicide for the analyst. Who benefits from the detective's labors? Not the criminal hiding the secret. The detective's job is to harm, not help, the criminal; in the process, he also helps himself and the society he protects from criminals. We see here how readily Freud assumes the traditional role of the psychiatrist as the protector of the community from the "dangerous madman."

Here, then, is the fly—nay, the elephant—in the ointment. Morelli's and Holmes's professional identities and duties are unambiguous: they are experts who detect and expose fakes/fakers and crimes/criminals; the exposed are devalued/punished. *Per analogiam*, what is Freud's professional identity and obligation? Is he a detector of secret malingerers/miscreants? If so, then his duty is to expose and punish them as fakers. Or is Freud a mental healer, a doctor of medicine whose duty is to help—never to harm—his patients? But if, as I maintain, his patients were not "ill" because there are no mental illnesses, then there are no treatments for them, psychoanalysis is not a (literal) treatment, and Freud did not (literally) treat patients.[29]

What was Freud—the self-defined expert on faking—exposing? He maintained that he was exposing the *erroneous explanation of hysteria as a counterfeit illness*. This exposure was necessary, he said, to make possible its replacement with the correct explanation of hysteria as a real illness, psychopathology.

Freud was playing a taxonomic shell game. In the conventional medical view, if the illness is fake, so too is the patient, the diagnosis, and the treatment. In Freud's interpretation, the "fakeness" in hysteria lies in attributing it to bodily (somatic) pathology instead of to mental (psycho) pathology. His explication leaves us with the following parallel: Morelli identifies forged artworks, Holmes solves baffling crimes, and Freud discovers the hidden psychological causes/determinants of psychogenic illnesses. But there are no similarities between crimes and the psychological causes of so-called mental (psychogenic) illnesses. Crimes are facts. Psychological causes and psychogenic diseases are fictions.

In the pre-Freudian scenario, malingering is self-created. In the post-Freudian scenario, it is still self-created but with this twist: it is caused by the "unconscious self" without the knowledge of the "conscious self." At one fell swoop, Freud "discovers" the cause of the illness and "cures" it. Both the discovery and the cure are frauds: there is no illness; hence, there is no cure.

V

Popular interest in the detection of art forgeries, detective stories, hysteria as a disease, and psychoanalysis as a theory and treatment started at about the same time, during the second half of the nineteenth century. Is there a connection among these seemingly disparate events, and, if so, what is it? Before answering that question, let me identify the principal dramatis personae.

Sigmund Freud (1856–1939) needs no introduction. Arthur Conan Doyle (1859–1930), born in Edinburgh, Scotland, to Irish Catholic parents, studied medicine at the University of Edinburgh, worked as a ship's doctor, and, in 1882, set up practice in Plymouth. Having hardly any patients, he began writing stories, introducing Sherlock Holmes to the public in 1887.

Dissatisfied with being a general practitioner, Doyle traveled to Vienna to study eye diseases and, in 1891, set up in London to practice as an ophthalmologist. Again, having few patients, he resumed writing. Eventually, Holmes appears in fifty-six short stories and four novels by Doyle, and in many more by other authors. A fervent advocate of justice, Doyle personally

investigated two cases leading to the release of the men wrongfully imprisoned. It should be noted that Doyle did not invent the genre of detective
fiction; he popularized it. Edgar Allan Poe (1809–1849), author of the
three famous Auguste Dupin tales—"The Murders in the Rue Morgue"
(1841), "The Mystery of Marie Roget" (1843), and "The Purloined Letter"
(1844)—was an important forerunner.

After the death of Doyle's wife in 1906, and the deaths of one of his
sons, his brother, his two brothers-in-law, and his two nephews in World War
I, Doyle became depressed and found solace in occultism and spiritualism.
Paradoxically, Doyle became an admirer and friend of the famous Hungarian
American magician Harry Houdini (Erich Weiss [1874–1926]), who was a
leading debunker of mediums and spiritualism, a conflict that eventually led
to the breakdown of their relationship.

Giovanni Morelli (1816–1891) was a Swiss Italian polymath: physician,
patriot, art historian, pioneer semiotician, and expert in distinguishing original artworks from imitations. Born in Verona to Swiss parents, with the birth
name Nicolas Schäffer, his first publications appeared under the pseudonym
Ivan Lermoliev. Morelli developed a method of observing artworks—systematically concentrating attention on seemingly minor details that revealed
the artist's typical modus operandi, such as his particular style of portraying
hands and ears—and based a scholarship in art forgery on it.

Morelli introduced his revolutionary views in the German art history
journal *Zeitschrift für bildende Kunst,* identifying himself as a Russian
scholar. The German translator, identified as Johannes Schwarze, was also
a fiction. Fluent in German, Morelli wrote the piece in German. Morelli's
major thesis was that the great European museums of art are full of fake
masterpieces, that is, paintings erroneously attributed to famous artists.

The connections between Freud, Doyle, and Morelli—all physicians
famous for works unrelated to medicine—were fruitfully analyzed by noted
Italian historian and semiotician Carlo Ginzburg (1939–): "In the following
pages, I will try to show how, in the late nineteenth century, an epistemological model (or, if you like, a paradigm) quietly emerged in the sphere of
the social sciences. Examining this paradigm, . . . which came into use without ever being spelled out as a theory, can perhaps help us to go beyond the
sterile contrasting of 'rationalism' and 'irrationalism.'"[30]

Ginzburg credits Italian art historian Enrico Castelnuovo with demonstrating the parallels between the method Conan Doyle attributed to Sherlock Holmes and Morelli's method of detecting art forgeries: each discovers, from clues unnoticed by others, the identity of a criminal or an artist. Freud, as noted, acknowledged Morelli's influence on his own work. Ginzburg explains the triple analogy by all three men having been trained in medicine "based on the interpretation of clues," and by tracing the origin of the use of small clues to mankind's prehistory, when survival depended on hunting:

> Hunters learned to reconstruct the appearance and movements of an unseen quarry through its tracks-prints in soft ground, snapped twigs, droppings, snagged hairs or feathers, smells, puddles, threads of saliva. They learned to sniff, to observe, to give meaning and context to the slightest trace. They learned to make complex calculations in an instant, in shadowy wood or treacherous clearing. Successive generations of hunters enriched and passed on this inheritance of knowledge. We have no verbal evidence to set beside their rock paintings and artifacts, but we can turn perhaps to the folktale, which sometimes carries an echo—faint and distorted—of what those far-off hunters knew. Three brothers (runs a story from the Middle East told among Kirghiz, Tatars, Jews, Turks, and so on) meet a man who has lost a camel (or sometimes it is a horse). At once they describe it to him: it's white, and blind in one eye; under the saddle it carries two skins, one full of oil, the other of wine. They must have seen it? No, they haven't seen it. So they're accused of theft and brought to be judged. The triumph of the brothers follows: they immediately show how from the barest traces they were able to reconstruct the appearance of an animal they had never set eyes on. . . . This "deciphering" and "reading" of animals' tracks is metaphorical. But it is worth trying to understand it literally, as the verbal distillation of a historical process leading, though across a very long time-span, toward the invention of writing.[31]

Ginzburg's learned essay abounds with brilliant insights into connections between diverse ways of seeing the world around us. One of these insights is the break between the concrete-individual-conjectural way of knowing and the abstract-general-mathematical way:

> Now it is clear that none—not even medicine—of the disciplines which
> we have been describing as conjectural would meet the criteria of scientific

inference essential to the Galilean [physicalistic-positivistic [*Naturwissen-schaftliches*], approach. They were above all concerned with the qualitative, the individual case or situation or document *as individual,* which meant there was always an element of chance in their results: one need only think of the importance of conjecture (a word whose Latin origin lies in divination) in medicine or philology, let alone in divination. Galilean [natural] science was altogether different; it could have taken over the scholastic saying "individuum est ineffable" (we can say nothing about the individual). Using mathematics and the experimental method involved the need to measure and to repeat phenomena, whereas an individualizing approach made the latter impossible and allowed the former only in part. All of which explains why historians have never managed to work out a Galilean method.[32]

It is important to note here that, thanks to advances in technology during the past half century, experts now distinguish forgeries from original works of art by objective methods, such as radiochemical identification of the chronological age of the painting or other art object, not by studying subtle clues of style. Similarly, so-called clinical diagnoses now rest on objective biochemical, radiological, and serological tests for identifying disease processes rather than subtle clues revealed by the patient's history and appearance. The practicing physician's experience and intuition, formerly called his "diagnostic acumen," have largely been replaced by objective evidence about the patient's biological health or illness. Such information—in contrast to the information gathered by persons engaged in the ideographic sciences *(Geisteswissenschaften)*—cannot easily be falsified by the parties concerned.

As I show in this book, deception and prevarication are the everyday tools of the detective, the psychologist, the psychiatrist, and the psychoanalyst. Freud's famous essay "The Moses of Michelangelo" (1914) is an example. Published anonymously, the piece was accompanied by a mendacious "explanatory note" that represented the writer as an "anonymous author whose mode of thought has in point of fact a certain resemblance to the methodology of psychoanalysis."[33] Freud waited ten years before revealing that he was the author and never adequately explained why he had lied about it.

Pseudoscience investigator Marcello Truzzi (1935–2003) correctly notes that Holmes was also not beyond the use of deception if he felt it might suit the ends of justice:

> Holmes was aware of the need to obtain the full confidence of his informants, and this he sometimes did by passing himself off as a groom, explaining to Watson, that "there is a wonderful sympathy and freemasonry among horsey men. Be one of them, and you will know all there is to know." On other occasions, Holmes faked illnesses, accidents, information, and even his own death. He often used the newspapers in a manipulative manner and noted that "the press . . . is a most valuable institution, if you only know how to use it."[34]

These observations alert us to the misleading aspects of the analogy between the physician diagnosing disease of the body and the detective diagnosing crime ("the disease of the body politic"), and, more important, to the differences between the physician diagnosing bodily disease and the psychoanalyst diagnosing mental disease. The radiologist does not need to gain the confidence of the patient to diagnose a skull fracture, and the pathologist does not need to gain the confidence of the corpse to make a postmortem diagnosis of death owing to drowning. In contrast, the psychoanalyst needs to gain the confidence of the patient to learn what ails him.

4 Sheltering

Confinement [in a mental hospital] has always been the greatest dread
of my life.

—Tennessee Williams (1911–1983), *Memoirs*

Two of our most important possessions—both characterized in the Declaration of Independence as "unalienable"—are the right to life and the right to liberty. It is impossible to overemphasize that psychiatry began with depriving certain individuals innocent of lawbreaking of liberty, that this practice still flourishes and forms the backbone of psychiatry, and that it is mendaciously called "hospitalization," not imprisonment. Carl Wernicke (1848–1905), one of the founders of modern neuropathology and neuropsychiatry, soberly noted that "the medical treatment of [mental] patients began with the infringement of their personal freedom."[1]

Fond of seeing themselves as bona fide physicians "saving lives," psychiatrists eagerly accepted the invitation of jurists to reduce the frequency of executions by declaring some criminals sentenced to death to be insane and therefore unfit to be punished. This practice, called the "insanity defense," also results in the incarceration of the offender, in a prison called a "mental hospital."[2] The insanity defense and civil commitment are psychiatry's two paradigmatic practices. Without them, (coercive) psychiatry would lose its social function and disappear.

Ever since the creation of insane asylums, some three hundred years ago, it has been common knowledge that individuals incarcerated in them were mistreated. In 1887, Nellie Bly, a young journalist, set out to write an exposé of the inhuman conditions to which the inmates of the Women's Lunatic Asylum in Manhattan were suspected of being subjected. She assumed the role of a pauper lunatic, had herself committed, and wrote an account of her experiences, published serially in the *New York Sun* and subsequently in book form. In those days, journalists and the public were not yet corrupted to know everything about mental illness that "ain't so": insane asylums were recognized as snake pits, not "hospitals"; journalists who set out to deceive psychiatrists were understood to be reporters, not "pseudopatients."

Bly's real name was Elizabeth Jane Cochran (1867–1922). She changed her name to Cochrane because she thought it was more elegant. While still in her teens, a sexist column in the *Pittsburgh Dispatch* prompted Cochrane to write a fiery rebuttal to it. The editor offered her a job and gave her the pen name "Nellie Bly."

Bly began her journalistic career at the *Dispatch* by writing a series of investigative articles about female factory workers. When barely twenty-one, she spent six months in Mexico as a foreign correspondent, her dispatches later published in book form as *Six Months in Mexico*. In 1887, when she was assigned to cover fashion, society, and gardening, the usual role for female reporters of the day, she quit her job, moved to New York City, and talked her way into being hired as a reporter for Joseph Pulitzer's sensationalist newspaper, the *New York World*.

It was Colonel John Cockerill, managing editor of the *World,* who proposed that Bly feign insanity, get herself committed to the Women's Lunatic Asylum on Blackwell's Island, and write an exposé of the institution.[3] The twenty-three-year-old Bly did it, wrote a powerful series of columns about her observations and experiences, and became an overnight sensation. She wrote, "Could I assume the characteristics of insanity to such a degree that I could pass the doctors, live for a week among the insane without the authorities there finding out that I was only a 'chiel [Scottish, lad] amang 'em takin' notes?' I said I believed I could. I had some faith in my own ability as an actress and thought I could assume insanity long enough to accomplish any mission intrusted to me."[4]

Bly speaks of having herself "committed to an insane asylum." In 1887, a person could not gain admission to an insane asylum by requesting it, just as he could not gain admission to prison by requesting it. To qualify as insane, the subject had to be an unwanted pauper. Bly emphasizes that the main challenge she faced was escaping detection. This assertion rests on an erroneous premise, namely, that the doctors were interested in distinguishing insane inmates properly committed from sane inmates falsely detained. The whole history of psychiatry belies this assumption. The presence of every inmate in an insane asylum affirmed the medical identity of the keepers as "doctors," and of the kept as "patients." Bly says that she

> always had a desire to know asylum life more thoroughly—a desire to be convinced that the most helpless of God's creatures, the insane, were cared for kindly and properly. The many stories I had read of abuses in such institutions I had regarded as wildly exaggerated. . . . I shuddered to think how completely the insane were in the power of their keepers, and how one could weep and plead for release, and all of no avail, if the keepers were so minded. Eagerly I accepted the mission to learn the inside workings of the Blackwell Island Insane Asylum. "How will you get me out," I asked my editor, "after I once get in?" "I do not know," he replied, "but we will get you out if we have to tell who you are, and for what purpose you feigned insanity."

Bly provides an excellent, down-to-earth account of how she pretended to be a lonely girl from Cuba lost in New York, penniless, unemployed, and unwanted. Assuming that role and acting crazy achieved her aim: she quickly found herself on Blackwell's Island.

> [I was committed to] the insane ward at Blackwell's Island, where I spent ten days and nights and had an experience which I shall never forget. I took upon myself to enact the part of a poor, unfortunate crazy girl, and felt it my duty not to shirk any of the disagreeable results that should follow. I became one of the city's insane wards for that length of time, experienced much, and saw and heard more of the treatment accorded to this helpless class of our population, and when I had seen and heard enough, my release was promptly secured. I left the insane ward with pleasure and regret—pleasure that I was once more able to enjoy the free breath of heaven; regret that I could not have brought with me some of the unfortunate women who lived and suffered with me, and who, I am convinced, are just as sane as I was and am now myself.

The die had been cast a hundred years earlier: some people were sane, others insane. Although each time experience was consulted, it showed that the experts were unable to distinguish the sane from the insane, each failure only confirmed the premise-as-conclusion. The reason is obvious: individuals become categorized as insane when they become troublesome to, and unwanted by, the people around them, and lack the power to resist being incarcerated in a madhouse. Bly observes the mistreatment of her fellow inmates and asserts her conviction that many of "the unfortunate women who lived and suffered with me . . . are just as sane as I was and am now myself." Yet she does not ask herself why, then, they continue to be confined. Who benefits from their confinement? Anticipating by a century the "scientific methods" of studies of the sanity-insanity conundrum, Bly emphasizes that "from the moment I entered the insane ward on the Island, I made no attempt to keep up the assumed *role* of insanity. I talked and acted just as I do in ordinary life. Yet strange to say, the more sanely I talked and acted the crazier I was thought to be." Bly quickly discovers that patients cannot possibly convince the doctors to set them free:

> I always made a point of telling the doctors I was sane and asking to be released, but the more I endeavored to assure them of my sanity the more they doubted it. . . . How can a doctor judge a woman's sanity by merely bidding her good morning and refusing to hear her pleas for release? . . . Again I said to one, "You have no right to keep sane people here. I am sane, have always been so and I must insist on a thorough examination or be released. Several of the women here are also sane. Why can't they be free?" "They are insane," was the reply, "and suffering from delusions." . . . The insane asylum on Blackwell's Island is a human rat-trap. It is easy to get in, but once there it is impossible to get out.

Bly's exposé resulted in an investigation of the asylum. She was summoned to testify, under oath, before the grand jury. "I answered the summons with pleasure, because I longed to help those of God's most unfortunate children whom I had left prisoners behind me. If I could not bring them that boon of all boons, liberty, I hoped at least to influence others to make life more bearable for them." The jurors requested that Bly accompany them on a visit to the island:

> I was glad to consent. No one was expected to know of the contemplated trip to the Island, yet we had not been there very long before one of the . . . jurors

told me that in conversation with a man about the asylum, he heard that they were notified of our coming an hour before we reached the Island. . . . The trip to the island was vastly different to my first. This time we went on a clean new boat, while the one I had traveled in, they said, was laid up for repairs. Some of the nurses were examined by the jury. . . . They confessed that the jury's contemplated visit had been talked over between them and the doctor. Dr. Dent confessed that . . . he knew the food was not what it should be, but said it was due to the lack of funds. . . . He said all the doctors were not competent, which was also due to the lack of means to secure good medical men. . . . The jurors then visited the kitchen. It was very clean. . . . The bread on exhibition was beautifully white and wholly unlike what was given us to eat. We found the halls in the finest order. The beds were improved. . . . *The institution was on exhibition, and no fault could be found.*

The grand jury duly recommended "improvements" and appropriated "$1,000,000 more than was ever before given for the benefit of the insane." Who benefited from these funds and the billions more that politicians have since then poured down the rat hole of institutional psychiatry? The psychiatrists and others employed by the asylum system. No one then in authority wanted to see, no one in authority wants to see, that psychiatric "reforms" are counterproductive. Chattel slavery needed to be abolished, not reformed. The same goes for psychiatric slavery.

I

In modern life, there are many situations in which society invites, as it were, psychiatrists to play the role of protecting people from certain perils. Protection from the perils of military service stands high on this list of psychiatric diagnosis as excuse-making. The first total war, based on the mobilization of the entire adult male populations of belligerent nations, was World War I. This war rendered the threat of conscription for military service a danger to men subject to the draft. Staying out of military service as well as trying to get out of it became powerful motives for malingering. In this situation, psychiatrists often assumed the roles of humanitarian doctors, diagnosing malingerers as suffering from hysteria, thus protecting them from the "death sentence" of having to return to the trenches.[5]

Before the war, the standard psychiatric treatment for hysteria was the so-called electric treatment, or "faradism," a procedure consisting of the application of interrupted DC (direct current) stimuli to the patient's supposedly affected muscles and nerves. Its effect, if any, was owing solely to suggestion. In his early years of practice, Freud routinely used this method. Its employment for the treatment of "war hysteria"—in other words, war neurosis, traumatic neurosis, shell shock, today anxiety, depression, and post-traumatic stress disorder—was an extension of this standard psychiatric therapy to military malingerers treated by doctors pretending to believe that the shirkers were sick.

On November 11, 1918, World War I formally ended, and the next day the Austro-Hungarian empire collapsed. Some veterans lost no time accusing medical officers of torturing them with painful electric currents in military psychiatric hospitals. Sensational charges in newspapers followed. The scandal quickly embroiled the most revered Austrian physician, Julius Wagner-Jauregg. Although only one person, named Walter Kauders, filed formal charges against him, and although Wagner-Jauregg was quickly and completely exonerated of any wrongdoing, his celebrity guaranteed that the affair would become a dramatic chapter in the history of psychiatry, specifically the history of malingering and hysteria-neurosis.

Julius Wagner-Jauregg (1857–1940) was a professor of psychiatry and neurology at the University of Vienna Medical School. He was the discoverer of iodine deficiency as the cause of cretinism (1884) and of fever treatment for neurosyphilis (1917), for which he received the Nobel Prize in Medicine in 1927. Though he remained a civilian, Wagner-Jauregg volunteered his services and used electrical treatment on patients diagnosed as suffering from war neuroses. In December 1918—barely one month after the cessation of hostilities—the provisional Austrian National Assembly appointed a commission to investigate the charges. The inquiry into Wagner-Jauregg's conduct—in which Freud gave expert testimony—became the centerpiece of the affair.

In 1985, Austrian American medical psychoanalyst Kurt R. Eissler published a meticulously researched account of the work of the commission investigating the accusations of "electrical torture" brought against Austrian military physicians in World War I, with special attention to the case of

Wagner-Jauregg. Born in Vienna, Eissler emigrated to the United States in 1938. After practicing psychoanalysis in Chicago and serving in the military during World War II, he established himself in New York and became one of the leaders of postwar psychoanalysis in the United States.

II

Virtually all of Eissler's work has as its principal aim the blindly zealous defense of the persona and work of Sigmund Freud. His book on the case against Wagner-Jauregg is no exception: it is titled *Freud as an Expert Witness: The Discussion of War Neuroses Between Freud and Wagner-Jauregg.* At the time of writing it, Eissler had lived in the United States for forty-seven years and had published extensively in English. Nevertheless, he wrote this work in German and credited the English translation, published in 1986, to a professional translator.

Eissler begins his book with an epigraph from the autobiography of Leopold Infeld (1898–1968), a Polish physicist and onetime colleague of Einstein: "I was a soldier in the Austro-Hungarian Army. . . . During these two years I malingered. I simulated diseases, forged identification papers, risked prison. . . . I did everything in my power to make Germany and Austria lose the war. In 1918, I thought myself to have been successful."[6]

Eissler acknowledges that writing *Freud as an Expert Witness* was an emotionally charged experience: "The themes of this book touch me very closely in a variety of respects. The principal actors, Wagner-Jauregg and Freud, are not, for me, figures of past history. Although I never met Freud, he is as much alive within me as though he were still with us."[7] Eissler loves Freud and despises Wagner-Jauregg. He is so prejudiced that he fails to mention that Freud and Wagner-Jauregg were friends. Approximately the same age, they were acquainted in medical school and addressed one another as *Du,* an important sign in the Vienna of those days of personal closeness.

Sixty years after the Wagner-Jauregg affair, Eissler meets Walter Kauders—the third dramatis persona in this Viennese passion play—in New York. Eissler does not say how the two met. He writes, "I had the good fortune to make the personal acquaintance in New York of Mr. Walter Kauders, who was at the center of the investigation against Wagner-Jauregg. . . . My account gains in depth from this lucky chance." Was this encounter a "lucky chance," or did Eissler, with his customary zeal for ferreting out details about all manner of events that touched Freud's life, seek out Kauders, the better to discredit Wagner-Jauregg? The evidence points in the latter direction. Eissler claims that he studied Kauders's case and concluded that Kauders had suffered a head injury and had been misdiagnosed and mistreated by Wagner-Jauregg and the other neurologists and psychiatrists with whom he had professional contact: "[Kauders's] mental health was beyond question, yet he was kept locked in a padded cell for months. In the adjoining cells were lunatics whose ceaseless howling prevented him from sleeping."[8] Eissler was a psychiatrist-psychoanalyst who saw mental illness wherever he looked. But when he looked at Kauders—who was not, let us remember, Eissler's patient, and Eissler never "examined" him—Eissler had no trouble concluding that Kauders was mentally healthy and had been wrongfully incarcerated.

The commission was presided over by Alexander Löffler (1866–1929), a Hungarian-born professor of law at the University of Vienna. He called on numerous physicians to present expert testimony, among them Freud, whom Eissler characterizes as an expert whose "work on the treatment of this group of illnesses [*sic*] led to important psychological discoveries and to the development of a new therapy; both became known all over the world as psychoanalysis."[9] Freud submitted a written memorandum to the commission, which is included in the *Standard Edition* and Eissler reprints in his book.[10] It is an extraordinarily arrogant and self-serving document that ends with this remarkable sentence: "But with the end of the war the war neurotics, too, disappeared—a final but impressive proof of the *psychical causation [Verursachung] of their illness.*"[11] In the memorandum, Freud offers this opinion about the electrical treatment of war neuroses:

> This insight into the causation of the war neuroses led to a method of treatment which seemed to be well-grounded and also proved to be highly effective in the first instance. *It seemed expedient to treat the neurotic as a malingerer and to disregard the psychological distinction between conscious and unconscious intentions, although he was not known to be a malingerer.* Since his illness served the purpose of withdrawing him from an intolerable situation, the roots of the illness would clearly be undermined if it was

made even more intolerable to him than active service. Just as he had fled from the war into illness, means were now adopted which compelled him to flee back from illness into health, that is to say, into fitness for active service. For this purpose painful electrical treatment was employed, and with success.[12]

In part, this explanation was intended as Freud's defense of Wagner-Jauregg's work. Ostensibly, all of it had something to do with illness and health, medicine and treatment. But it did not. Malingerers faked illness and played the roles of disabled patients. Doctors faked treatment and played the roles of morally neutral, scientific healers. It was one fraud complemented by another fraud. To make his point with regard to Wagner-Jauregg clear, Freud adds, "If [the electrical treatment] was used in the Vienna Clinics [of Wagner-Jauregg], *I am personally convinced that it was never intensified to a cruel pitch at the initiative of Professor Wagner-Jauregg.* I cannot vouch for other physicians whom I did not know."[13]

Freud had no firsthand knowledge of what was taking place in Austrian military hospitals. His testimony was wholly hearsay, of no probative value in a legal investigation. Called to testify as an expert, the honorable thing would have been to decline the invitation to testify about accusations brought against physicians about whose work he had no firsthand knowledge. Instead, Freud seized the opportunity to puff psychoanalysis and advance his professional position by exonerating his famous colleague. He continues, "The psychological education of medical men is in general decidedly deficient and more than one of them may have forgotten that the *patient whom he was seeking to treat as a malingerer was, after all, not one.*" Freud concludes by complimenting himself: "In 1918, Dr. Ernst Simmel [a psychoanalyst disciple] . . . published a pamphlet in which he reported the *extraordinarily favorable results achieved in severe cases of war neurosis by the psychotherapeutic method introduced by me.*"[14]

In his memorandum, Freud states, "Thus the precondition of the war neuroses would seem to be a national [conscript] army; there would be no possibility of their arising in an army of professional soldiers or mercenaries." So much for Freud's insights into economics, politics, and human nature. Regarding the differences between malingering and hysteria, Freud explains,

"The soldier in whom these affective motives were very powerful and clearly conscious would . . . have been obliged to desert or pretend to be ill. Only the smallest proportion of war neurotics, however, were malingerers; the emotional impulses which rebelled in them . . . were operative in them without becoming conscious to them."[15] In the Austro-Hungarian army, viewed through the all-seeing eyes of Sigmund Freud, rebellions were staged by "unconscious emotional impulses," not rebellious soldiers.

III

In 1972, David L. Rosenhan, then a young psychologist, undertook to stage a psychiatric impersonation similar to the one staged by Bly almost a century before. He defined his hoax as a scientific experiment, called the hoaxers "pseudopatients," decked out his account as a scholarly study, and had it published, to great acclaim, in *Science,* the most respected American scientific journal, under the title "On Being Sane in Insane Places."[16] In the mental health literature, the piece is typically referred to as the "pseudopatient study."

We have a choice among several terms with which to identify the person who pretends to be mad: the terms we choose prejudge and may largely determine the inferences we draw from the reports of the patient-doctor encounter. Bly assumed the mad role qua journalist, to write an exposé. Today, she would be called an "investigative journalist." A soldier who malingers, as Bly did, would now be regarded as suffering from PTSD and compensated for his "service-connected injury." Rosenhan defined himself as a "pseudopatient," an academic scholar engaged in pioneering psychiatric research. This self-description is objectionable. Consider the following cases: Authors who appropriate passages from the works of other authors are not pseudowriters; they are real writers we call "plagiarists." Painters who imitate the works of famous artists are not pseudopainters; they are real painters we call "forgers." Psychologists who impersonate the role of mental patients are not pseudopatients; they are real patients, "forgers" of the mad role. They are pseudoinsane, not pseudopatients.

Each of these actors has his own motives. Each is a dramatis personae in a real-life drama. None is sick, and none is a scientist. When a person asserts that he is not who he is, and claims that he is, say, Jesus, psychiatrists diagnose him as suffering from a severe form of mental illness and diagnose him as schizophrenic. Elsewhere, I have proposed viewing this phenomenon as a type of "identity theft." The schizophrenic and the identity thief both know who they are.

I consider Rosenhan's calling himself a "pseudopatient" a type of "lying truth," a variation on the theme of counterfeiting mental illness and engaging in a duplicitous "dance" with the psychiatric establishment.[17] Rosenhan does not examine, much less challenge, the concept of mental illness. On the contrary, frequently using the legalistic term *insanity* instead of the "medical" term *mental illness,* he writes:

> If sanity and insanity exist, how shall we know them? . . . To raise questions regarding normality and abnormality is in no way to question the fact that some behaviors are deviant or odd. Murder is deviant. So, too, are hallucinations. Nor does raising such questions deny the existence of the personal anguish that is often associated with "mental illness." Anxiety and depression exist. Psychological suffering exists. But normality and abnormality, sanity and insanity, and the diagnoses that flow from them may be less substantive than many believe them to be.

Asking, as Rosenhan asks, "If sanity and insanity exist, how shall we know them?" is disingenuous. For more than a decade before Rosenhan published his paper, I argued that mental illness is a fiction, a metaphor. This contention was widely discussed in both the popular press and the professional literature. Rosenhan pretends to believe that sanity and insanity exist; the only question is, "how shall we know them?" Undaunted, he continues:

> At its heart, the question of whether the sane can be distinguished from the insane . . . is a simple matter: Do the salient characteristics that lead to *diagnoses* reside in the patients themselves or in the environments and contexts in which observers find them? From Bleuler, through Kretchmer, through the formulators of the recently revised *Diagnostic and Statistical Manual* of the American Psychiatric Association, the belief has been strong that patients present symptoms, that those symptoms can be categorized, and, implicitly, that the sane are distinguishable from the insane.

Rosenhan knows and acknowledges that "belief [in mental illness] has been questioned" but, comme il faut, does not mention my name or refer to my writings. Instead, he assumes that psychiatrists cannot distinguish the sane from the insane and grandly asserts, "This article describes such an experiment. . . . Eight sane people gained secret admission to 12 different hospitals. Their diagnostic experiences constitute the data of the first part of this article." The sane people, whom Rosenhan calls "pseudopatients," *did not "gain admission": they went to emergency rooms, lied to psychiatrists that they were hearing voices, and in effect asked to be admitted to their hospitals.* Rosenhan's language contains his conclusion: "After calling the hospital for an appointment, the pseudopatient arrived at the admissions office complaining that he had been hearing voices. Asked what the voices said, he replied that they were often unclear, but as far as he could tell they said 'empty,' 'hollow,' and 'thud.' . . . The choice of these symptoms was occasioned by their apparent similarity to existential symptoms . . . and the absence of a single report of existential psychoses in the literature."

The persons who arrived at the hospital were self-defined mental patients, not pseudopatients. Their con game is evident, albeit Rosenhan befogs it with psychobabble. At the same time, the foregoing vignette illustrates how successfully Rosenhan had been indoctrinated into the role of a clinical psychologist and how eagerly and uncritically he embraced the dehumanized ("delusional") ideology and vocabulary of that cult. One person, ostensibly seeking professional help, says, "I hear a voice that says 'thud.'" The other person, instead of saying something like, "Why are you telling me this? What do you want me to do about it?" concludes that his interlocutor has schizophrenia and incarcerates him. Rosenhan then spins this minidrama of psychiatric impersonation into a "scientific" article that *Science* publishes as a signal contribution to the science of psychiatry. Rosenhan continues, "Immediately upon admission to the psychiatric ward, the pseudopatient ceased simulating any symptoms of abnormality. . . . [T]he pseudopatient behaved on the ward as he 'normally' behaved. . . . Despite their public 'show' of sanity, the pseudopatients were never detected. Admitted, except in one case, with a diagnosis of schizophrenia, each was discharged with a diagnosis of schizophrenia 'in remission.'"

Along the way, Rosenhan discovers that "what holds for medicine does not hold equally well for psychiatry. Medical illnesses, while unfortunate,

are not commonly pejorative. Psychiatric diagnoses, on the contrary, carry
with them personal, legal, and social stigmas. . . . Having once been labeled
schizophrenic, there is nothing the pseudopatient can do to overcome the
tag." We did not need Rosenhan's study to learn this point.

Although Rosenhan's essay is relatively brief, it is, for anyone familiar
with the history of psychiatry, full of platitudes: "A psychiatric label has a
life and an influence of its own. Once the impression has been formed that
the patient is schizophrenic, the expectation is that he will continue to be
schizophrenic. . . . Eventually, the patient himself accepts the diagnosis, with
all of its surplus meanings and expectations, and behaves accordingly." None
of this discussion is new.

Lest the right-thinking psychiatrist or psychologist mistakenly regard
the "pseudopatient study" as a psychiatric exposé, Rosenhan repeatedly
reaffirms that he is a friend, not a foe, of the coercive-psychiatric establishment. He explains, "The term 'mental illness' [*sic,* not insanity] is of recent
origin. It was coined by people who were humane in their inclinations and
who wanted very much to raise the station of (and the public's sympathies
toward) the psychologically disturbed from that of witches and 'crazies' to
one that was akin to the physically ill. And they were at least partially successful, for the treatment of the mentally ill has improved considerably over
the years." These statements are all substantially untrue. After each declaration of loyalty to psychiatry, Rosenhan offers a familiar criticism, devoid of
shock value, such as the following:

> The patient is deprived of many of his legal rights by dint of his psychiatric
> commitment. He is shorn of credibility by virtue of his psychiatric label.
> His freedom of movement is restricted. He cannot initiate contact with the
> staff, but may only respond to such overtures as they make. Personal privacy
> is minimal. Patient quarters and possessions can be entered and examined
> by any staff member, for whatever reason. His personal history and anguish
> is available to any staff member (often including the "grey lady" and "candy
> striper" volunteer) who chooses to read his folder, regardless of their thera-
> peutic relationship to him. His personal hygiene and waste evacuation are
> often monitored. The water closets have no doors. . . . All told, the pseu-
> dopatients were administered nearly 2100 pills, including Elavil, Stelazine,
> Compazine, and Thorazine.

Rosenhan claims that out of twenty-one hundred pills, only two were swallowed, with the rest pocketed or flushed down the toilet. Is this report
believable? We are not told why those two pills were swallowed instead of
also being secreted.

Finally, Rosenhan rediscovers psychiatry's oldest problem, "false commitment": "How many people, one wonders, are sane but not recognized
as such in our psychiatric institutions?" He thus reinforces the legitimacy of
depriving people of dignity and liberty, provided they *really have real mental illnesses*. His premise reeks of the odor of bad faith. Rosenhan identifies
himself and his fellow frauds as sane pseudopatients and the other inmates in
the hospital as insane "real" patients, even though the latter were diagnosed
as insane by the same psychiatrists whose inability to make such a diagnosis
Rosenhan claims to have demonstrated.

After looking psychiatric coercion—a moral and political, not a medical,
issue—squarely in the eye, Rosenhan pretends to have not seen it and averts
his gaze. "I do not," he writes, "understand this problem well enough to
perceive solutions." Rosenhan sees no solution because he does not see that
the problem is coercion, and if the problem is coercion—that is, psychiatric slavery—then the only solution is its abolition. Instead, Rosenhan—like
Bly—sees promise in *expanding psychiatry:* "But two matters seem to have
some promise. The first concerns the proliferation of community mental
health facilities, of crisis intervention centers, of the human potential movement, and of behavior therapies. . . . Clearly, to the extent that we refrain
from sending the distressed to insane places, our impressions of them are less
likely to be distorted." Gorbachev saw nothing wrong with communism that
putting a "human face" on it could not remedy. The apparatchiks were fine,
upright persons needing only some "sensitivity training":

> Clearly, further research into the social psychology of such total institu-
> tions will both facilitate treatment and deepen understanding. . . . I and
> the other pseudopatients in the psychiatric setting had distinctly negative
> reactions. . . . It could be a mistake, and a very unfortunate one, to consider
> that what happened to us derived from malice or stupidity on the part of
> the staff. Quite the contrary, our overwhelming impression of them was of
> people who really cared, who were committed and who were uncommonly

intelligent. . . . Simply reading materials in this area will be of help to some such workers and researchers.

IV

Rosenhan claimed that he wanted to investigate whether psychiatrists and psychologists could "distinguish the sane from the insane." This assertion was a lie. Rosenhan knew that they could not be (objectively) distinguished because there are no hematological, histological, radiological, or other "real" medical tests for "insanity." He knew that the terms *sane* and *insane* are value judgments, like *beautiful* and *ugly*, not biological states, like *alive* and *dead*. Understanding what is wrong with Rosenhan's study—like understanding everything psychiatrists and psychologists write—requires paying close attention to his language. I emphasized earlier that Rosenhan called himself and his colleagues "pseudopatients" and that I consider this claim to be a deception. We don't call a fake Renoir that we know is a forgery a "pseudo-Renoir." As long as such a canvas passes as an original masterpiece, *it is a real Renoir*. Exposed as a fake, it is not a Renoir at all.

Rosenhan successfully impersonated a mental patient. He was a *real patient, not a pseudopatient:* mental illness stands in the same relation to bodily illness as a fake Renoir stands to a real Renoir.[18] Rosenhan removed the prefix from illness and attached it to the patient role. Being a patient is a role: the term has meaning only in the context of a particular relationship. Robinson Crusoe may have diabetes, but could not be a patient. Rosenhan understood this point. In his textbook (coauthored with Martin E. P. Seligman), he writes, "Thomas Szasz is one of the most critical analysts of the nature of psychiatry and its role in society today. Szasz points out that mental illness is different from physical illness. There are no clear or generally accepted criteria of mental illness. . . . 'Looking for evidence of such illness is like searching for evidence of heresy. Once the investigator gets into the proper frame of mind, anything may seem to him to be a symptom of mental illness' [citing *Law, Liberty, and Psychiatry* (1963)]." A few pages later Rosenhan cites my warning of the power of psychiatrists and psychologists and the danger posed by their alliance with the government in the therapeutic state (1963).[19] In 1979, in response to Rosenhan's so-called pseudopatient study, I wrote:

> With the growth of psychiatric research in the modern era, deception—long the stock-in-trade of the mental patient and the mental healer—became a favorite methodological device of the psychiatric investigator as well. . . . For example, in 1972, Dr. David Rosenhan and his associates set out to deliberately deceive a number of hospital psychiatrists. . . . Pretending to be hearing voices, they called mental hospitals and gained admission to them on the basis of that complaint. . . . This deception was supposedly necessitated by the problem to be investigated. "However distasteful such *concealment* is, it was a necessary first step to examining these questions," explained Rosenhan. . . . *But this experiment was not premised on concealment (as are double-blind studies), but rather on deception:* the researchers impersonated psychotics and deliberately lied to the psychiatrists whose help they ostensibly solicited. Nevertheless, not only was this study accepted for publication in *Science,* it was hailed as an important piece of research, supposedly proving the "labeling theory" of mental illness and the "unreliability" of the psychiatric-diagnostic process. To me it proved only that it is easy to deceive people, especially when they don't expect to be deceived.[20]

Disguising oneself to gain entry into forbidden territory, with the intention of damaging or destroying an adversary, is an ancient motif. Persons in charge of total institutions, housing inmates deprived of liberty and presumably ill-treated, carefully guard their turf against trespassers. Insane asylums, surrounded by high walls or other symbols of separation from society at large, have long been viewed as shadowy places of unspeakable horrors and secret indignities. This imagery has encouraged journalists to infiltrate and expose them, ostensibly in order to "reform" the "system." Such a stratagem, especially when employed to expose conditions in mental hospitals, suffers from a fatal flaw: the investigation is premised on the legitimacy of the institution and aims only to ameliorate or abolish its so-called abuses. In practice, the exposé reauthenticates the reality of mental illnesses, relegitimates the psychiatrist's power over the psychiatric inmate, and, in the process, distracts attention from the root problem that Roy Porter aptly termed "the conventions of insanity": "Properly speaking, contends Szasz, insanity is not a disease with origins to be excavated, but a behavior with meanings to be decoded. Social existence is a rule-governed game-playing ritual in which the mad person bends the rules and exploits the loopholes. Since the mad person is engaged in social performances that obey certain expectations so as to defy others, the pertinent questions are not about the origins, but about the conventions, of insanity."[21]

V

Rosenhan's impersonation of mental patients was published in the prestigious journal *Science* in 1973. It illustrated the absurdities of the psychiatric diagnostic process and became famous as the "pseudopatient study." The same year Donald Naftulin—a young psychiatrist at the University of Southern California at Los Angeles—hired an actor to impersonate a psychiatrist. His report illustrated the absurdities of the psychiatric educational process and was published in the obscure *Journal of Medical Education*.[22] It was not called the "pseudopsychiatrist study" and sank without a trace.

Naftulin and his collaborators hired a distinguished-looking professional actor, named him Dr. Myron L. Fox, bestowed upon him the persona of "an authority on the application of mathematics to human behavior," created a bogus curriculum vitae, coached him in a speech titled "Mathematical Game Theory as Applied to Physician Education," and asked him to deliver his lecture "charismatically and non-substantively." The "Dr. Fox Lecture" was first presented to a group of eleven psychiatrists, psychologists, and social work educators and was videotaped. The tape was then shown to another group of eleven psychiatrists, psychologists, and psychiatric social workers, and finally to a group of thirty-three educators and administrators taking a graduate course in educational philosophy. All fifty-five subjects were asked to answer a questionnaire evaluating their response to the lecture. The result was predictable: the pseudopsychiatrist was rated an outstanding psychiatrist: "All respondents had significantly more favorable than unfavorable responses. . . . One even believed he [had] read Dr. Fox's publications." A typical response was: "Excellent presentation, enjoyed listening . . . Good analysis of the subject . . . Knowledgeable." Naftulin concludes, "[The] study supports the possibility of training actors to give legitimate lectures as an innovative educational approach toward student-perceived satisfaction with the learning process."[23] Evidently, Naftulin saw nothing wrong with transforming an ostensibly educational event into a deliberate con game. This deception is consistent with his role as psychiatrist, a member of a special group of "actors." Psychiatrists are physicians who impersonate physicians: they *possess legitimate medical credentials but neither know real medicine nor practice as real medical doctors.* Because law and society regard their performances as useful, indeed indispensable, the fact that the soul doctors are fake doctors is generally disbelieved and disbelievable (except by persons who arrive at this conclusion by their own intellectual efforts, for whom it is obvious).

Actually, Rosenhan's and Naftulin's experiments were similar. Each showed that psychiatry qua medical specialty is nonsense, authenticated as common sense by society and its democratically chosen guardians. Neither was willing to risk his career by "denying the reality of mental illness." The psychiatrist's and the psychologist's professional identity depends on his authenticating mental illness as a disease like any other. The layperson is perhaps even more impeded in repudiating the psychiatric mythology: he hears about mental illness incessantly and "sees" mental illness wherever he looks. How can he be expected to believe that mental illness does not exist, that psychiatry is pseudology?

Recently, Gert Postel (1958–), a German postal worker, achieved a measure of mostly local fame for his successful impersonation of a psychiatrist. Angry at the psychiatric establishment for incarcerating and mistreating his mother and blaming her suicide on her treatment, Postel was not interested in studying psychiatry. He was interested in mocking it and unmasking its medical pretensions.

In 1995, having forged some medical documents, Postel obtained a position as senior physician in a psychiatric clinic in a Leipzig suburb. He lectured, provided psychiatric expert testimony to the courts, and was slated to be appointed to a professorship and the position of chief of medicine at Saxony's hospital for psychiatry and neurology at Arnsdorf, near Dresden. Postel's meteoric rise in the world of institutional psychiatry came crashing down, however, when, in 1997, a coworker recognized him. Postel went into hiding and was arrested, tried, convicted, and jailed in 1998, and released on probation in 2001. His exploits made him famous and notorious. In 2001 he published the story of his psychiatric impersonation, titled *Doktorspiele: Geständnisse eines Hochstaplers* (Playing Doctor: Confessions of a Confidence Man). The book was a best-seller in Germany.

Something of a celebrity, Postel has given numerous television interviews, most recently in 2007: "A world congress of psychiatrists in Dresden [in 2007] now once again prods the 48 year-old into action. 'All hot air there!,' according to Postel. . . . 'I introduced disease terms which do not even exist, e.g. the bipolar depression of the third degree, in front of 120 psychiatrists and not a single one dared to ask a question. . . . As far as Psychiatry is concerned it can be said that if you're able to perform linguistic acrobatics you can make a career for yourself. That is what Psychiatry is based on.'" Asked how he had obtained his job in the Leipzig clinic, Postel explained: "The chairman asked me: 'What did you write your doctorate about?' and I replied: 'About cognitive induced distortions of the stereotyped judgement formation.' That is a lining up of empty terms." Postel concludes, "The maliciousness of psychiatry is that it promotes itself as a medical discipline, although it is actually only part of the state authority."[24] Therein lies its power and its immunity to mockery by the powerless.

5 Cheating

He'll cheat without scruple, who can without fear.
—Benjamin Franklin (1706–1790)

In November 2007, German Olympic pole-vaulter Yvonne Buschbaum announced that she is retiring from track and field and "will become a man. . . . I feel as if I am a man and have to live my life in the body of a woman." Gender reassignment involves taking hormones that are on the World Anti-Doping Agency's list of banned substances. Buschbaum stated that "she has not taken any performance-enhancing drugs during her athletic career. 'I do not dope,' she said."[1]

Doped athleticism is fake athleticism; doped sex change is genuine treatment. This view is, of course, a new cultural convention, owing in part to the discovery of sex hormones, and in part to the secularization and medicalization of gender roles. And so also is our modern, secularized-medicalized perspective on faked illness.

I have long maintained that the phenomena conventionally called "mental illnesses" are counterfeit illnesses authenticated as genuine diseases by psychiatrists. The phenomenon, as we have seen, is not unique to mental illness. Not only do medical and legal authorities validate transgender males as females, and vice versa, they also validate self-killing (formerly "self-murder") as "wrongful death" owing to medical negligence, not the voluntary act of the self-killer.[2] Let us now reconsider the most instructive model of mental illness as validated counterfeit illness—the identification-validation of a forged masterpiece as an original masterpiece by art experts.

A forged masterpiece, authenticated as an original, is valuable. Exposed as a forgery, it becomes a worthless fake. Largely because of this elementary

economic-social fact, art collectors and museums must distinguish original works of art from forgeries. The same principle compels individuals and
institutions charged with the duty of caring and paying for medical services
to distinguish real diseases-patients from fake diseases-patients, that is, distinguish persons who harbor real diseases and occupy the patient role validly
from persons who do not harbor real diseases and occupy the patient role
nevertheless.

The story of Dutch master forger Han van Meegeren (1889–1947) provides the perfect model for a critical examination and correct understanding
of mental illnesses as medically and psychiatrically validated diseases. So
successful was van Meegeren that his forgeries, classified as original masterpieces, almost cost him his life: in the end, he had to expose himself as
a forger.[3]

I

Van Meegeren was a painter, art restorer, and the most famous art forger
of the twentieth century, perhaps of all time. A gifted artist, he became,
while still in his twenties, a successful portrait painter and a wealthy man.
His aspiration to become recognized as an artist on a par with the Dutch
masters was frustrated, however, by critics who denigrated his style as old-
fashioned. Embittered, van Meegeren decided to forge paintings by famous
artists. He spent six years studying the canvases, paints, brushes, and strokes
used by the masters whose works he decided to imitate. He created a mixture
of phenol and formaldehyde to cause the paints to harden after application,
making the paintings appear to be three hundred years old. After complet-
ing a painting, he baked it to dry, rolled a drum over it to crack it a little, and
washed it in black india ink to fill in the cracks. He produced such perfect
imitations of the works of Frans Hals (ca. 1581–1666), Pieter de Hooch
(1629–after 1684), Gerard ter Borch (1617–1681), and Johannes (Jan) Vermeer (1632–1675) that the best art experts and critics of the time declared
them genuine. He was, in his own mind at least, vindicated: his pictures
hung in museums and were celebrated throughout the world.

During World War II, wealthy Dutchmen, wanting to prevent Dutch
art from falling into the hands of the Nazis, avidly bought his forged

"originals." Nevertheless, one of van Meegeren's fake Vermeers ended up in the possession of Hermann Göring, who—compounding the ironies—had paid for it with counterfeit currency. Göring showcased the Vermeer forgery at his residence in Karinhall, north of Berlin. In August 1943, his paintings, including the "Vermeer" and thousands of other pieces of artwork looted by the Nazis, were stored in an Austrian salt mine, where, in May 1945, they were found by Allied troops. The fake Vermeer was eventually traced to van Meegeren. He was arrested and charged with "selling Dutch cultural property" to the Nazis, a crime punishable by death. Van Meegeren "confessed" that the "Vermeer" was a forgery and that he was the forger. No one believed him: prominent art experts unanimously testified that Göring's "Vermeer" was an original.

Imprisoned, van Meegeren asked the authorities to let him prove that he could paint "Vermeers." He was provided the art supplies he requested and between July and September 1945—in the presence of six witnesses, including a Vermeer expert, a photographer, and four police officers—painted his last forgery, a magnificent canvas he called *Jesus among the Doctors*.

Before proceeding with the trial, the court commissioned an international group of experts to address the authenticity of van Meegeren's paintings. The commission included curators and professors from the Netherlands, Belgium, and England and was led by Paul Coremans, director of the chemical laboratory at the Belgian Royal Museums of Fine Arts. Over a two-year period, the commission examined the Vermeer and Frans Hals paintings that van Meegeren had designated as forgeries. Coremans found that van Meegeren had prepared the paints by mixing modern white lead with a phenol-formaldehyde resin, both materials introduced and manufactured in the twentieth century.

Tried on November 12, 1947, van Meegeren was convicted of "falsification and fraud" and sentenced to one year in prison. Six weeks later he suffered a fatal heart attack, escaping having to serve his sentence. In a Dutch opinion poll after the war, van Meegeren was chosen as one of the most admired persons in the country.

Debate about the authenticity of van Meegeren's forgeries continued after his death and did not end until 1967. In 1951, Jean Decoen, a Brussels art expert and restorer, wrote a book in which he asserted that two of van

Meegeren's most famous paintings, *The Disciples at Emmaus* and *The Last Supper II*, were genuine Vermeers and claimed that the conclusions of Paul Coremans's panel of experts were wrong. He urged that the paintings be reexamined. Daniel George van Beuningen, a wealthy ship owner who had bought these pictures, demanded that Coremans publicly admit that he had erred in his analysis of van Meegeren's paintings. When Coremans refused, van Beuningen sued, alleging that Coremans's wrongful branding of the paintings diminished their value and asked for compensation in the amount of five hundred thousand pounds (about ten million dollars today). In May 1955, before the case came to trial, van Beuningen died. Seven months later, the court heard the case on behalf of van Beuningen's heirs and found in favor of Coremans, upholding the findings of his commission.

Finally, in 1967, the Artists Material Center at Carnegie Mellon University in Pittsburgh examined several of the "Vermeers" in their collection by measuring the radioactive decay of lead in white-lead pigments. They discovered that these paintings, too, were van Meegeren's forgeries. In the process, the experts confirmed the findings of the 1946 Coremans commission and refuted the claims made by Jean Decoen.

The van Meegeren affair illustrates the tragicomic consequences of forged masterpieces being authenticated as genuine. Psychiatry rests squarely on forged diseases being systematically authenticated as genuine and treated as real diseases: both "patients" and "doctors"—persons who define their dis-eases as illnesses and who define and diagnose problems in living as mental illnesses—are disease counterfeiters. The results of this orgy of medical counterfeiting are: (1) "disease museums," like the APA's *Diagnostic and Statistical Manuals,* full of forged diseases; (2) an expanding "mental health market," offering increasing numbers of drugs and other therapies for mental diseases, consuming increasing amounts of public and private resources; and (3) a growing number of professional disease forgers becoming more influential and wealthy.

II

I formed the idea that psychiatry was medical counterfeiting when I was quite young. Much later, I decided to qualify as a psychoanalytic psychiatrist to be in a position to analyze and address the subject intelligently and with authority.[4] In 1960, I published my paper "The Myth of Mental Illness" and, a year later, my book with the same title. These and some of my later writings, especially *The Manufacture of Madness,* undermined the medical legitimacy of the notion that mental illnesses—that is, behaviors not attributable to bodily lesions—are diseases, and generated a reaction revealingly called the "remedicalization of psychiatry." There is considerable psychiatric literature on this subject. Typically, remedicalization is defined as "the refocusing of scientific advances in neurobiology and neuroscience as they affect psychiatric diagnosis and treatment, increased psychiatrist involvement in the treatment of the physically ill and in organized medicine."[5]

The zeal for remedicalization culminates in physicians claiming all of human life for a medicalized psychiatry and psychiatrized medicine, epitomized by a demand for the abolition of the term *mental illness* and the quasi-theological faith in the claim that all mental illnesses are, *eo ipso,* brain diseases. Mary Baker, president of the European Parkinson's Disease Association, and Matthew Menken, World Federation of Neurology liaison representative to the World Health Organization, state:

> It is harmful to millions of people to declare that some brain disorders are not physical ailments. By 2020, diseases arising from nervous system disorders will make up 14.7% of all diseases worldwide (up from 10.5% in 1990), according to the Global Burden of Disease (GBD) Study recently carried out by the World Health Organization and other institutions. Although nervous system disorders comprise only 1.4% of all deaths, this study estimated that they account for a remarkable 28% of all years of life lived with a disability. Moreover, *much of the burden of illness due to road traffic incidents, violence, war, and falls is a consequence of nervous system dysfunction. The president of the World Federation of Neurology, James F. Toole, has highlighted brain dysfunction among world leaders as one of the greatest threats to global peace, and therefore the health of populations.*[6]

To perceive, define, and treat deviant behaviors as diseases and disliked persons as sick patients is, of course, (re)medicalization, pure and simple.[7] It is also mendacity on a grand scale and the source of psychiatric cheating on a scale to match. The assumption that mental illnesses are as yet undiscovered brain diseases liberates the biological psychiatrist from having to know his patient as a person. It is enough for him to know that the patient has been diagnosed as suffering from a mental illness, as it is (almost) enough for the surgeon to know that his patient has acute appendicitis. The "knowledge" that the patient has a brain disease justifies the psychiatrist to treat the patient *as if* he has a brain disease and treat him, if need be, without his consent and against his will. In a recent review of the concept of mental illness, psychologist Guy A. Boysen writes:

> Szasz correctly states that once objective biological signs are found, disorders stop being mental illnesses and become medical illnesses. Epilepsy, general paresis, and various medically caused cognitive disorders stand out as examples of the conversion of mental into physical illness. Reflecting the essentialist viewpoint, some have argued that the term mental illness should be eliminated because so-called mental illnesses are all brain disorders. The irony of reframing Szasz's claim that mental illness is a myth in its converse has not been lost on commentators.[8]

For most people today, there is nothing ironic about reframing the myth of mental illness as a huge error: today "we know" that all mental illnesses are brain diseases. The therapeutic state—the alliance of medicine and the state—has so decreed:

• *White House Fact Sheet on Myths and Facts about Mental Illness* (1999): "Research in the last decade proves that mental illnesses are diagnosable disorders of the brain."

• President William Jefferson Clinton (1999): "Mental illness can be accurately diagnosed, successfully treated, just as physical illness."

• Tipper Gore, President Clinton's mental health adviser (1999): "One of the most widely believed and most damaging myths is that mental illness is not a physical disease. Nothing could be further from the truth."

• Surgeon General David Satcher (1999): "Just as things go wrong with the heart and kidneys and liver, so things go wrong with the brain."

• Nancy C. Andreasen, professor of psychiatry at the University of Iowa (1997): "What we call 'mind' is the expression of the activity of the brain."[9]

The view that depression and schizophrenia are brain diseases is past debate or discussion: it is a collective article of psychiatric faith, protected and promoted by the power and the purse of the pharmacratic state. One unsurprising result is that the person labeled as a "psychiatric researcher" becomes the corrupt agent of the therapeutic state: he resembles the corrupt district attorney who, suspecting that the person charged with a crime may be innocent, perceives his job as having to fabricate evidence of his guilt. This deceit is what many psychiatrists claiming to have discovered evidence that schizophrenia is owing to a biological defect have done and continue to do. The work of the late Richard J. Wyatt (1939–2002), longtime chief of the neuropsychiatry branch at the National Institute of Mental Health (NIMH), illustrates this approach to solving the riddle of mental illness.

III

Wyatt was married to Kay Redfield Jamison, a psychologist, self-defined manic-depressive, and expert on "bipolar disease" and its biological-coercive treatment. Like his wife, Wyatt had a penchant for identifying himself in psychiatric terms. In an autobiographical essay, he stated:

> As far as I could tell, I had no visible talents. I had missed out on the genes for memory and rhythm. I was tone deaf. I could not draw. And though the term was not popular back then, I was (and am) dyslexic. . . . Around the same time, the discovery of Lloyd Castle Douglas's Doctor Hudson's Secret Journal combined with an uneasy adolescence to produce an enduring fascination with the brain. My head, limbs, and emotions had apparently lost all connection. . . . Yet even at thirteen, Douglas's divide between mind and brain struck me as pragmatic but not terribly interesting, with the result that his neurosurgeon hero gripped my imagination more spiritually than scientifically. I began reading everything I could about psychology. . . . I read about Mesmerism, hypnotism, and Freud. . . . My interest was piqued, but I concluded that psychodynamics—psychiatry's enchantment at the time—had become overextended in its effort to explain all of humanity. I found the tales of heavy-handed Freudianism emanating from the University of Chicago's Orthogenic School disturbing. . . . At any

rate, sitting passive and still has never been my strong suit. Some attention deficit disorder is mixed in with my dyslexia. . . . When it came time for college I chose the University of Michigan because of its size. I figured that I could manage the multiple-choice exams then used to test classes of a thousand or more students at a time. Unfortunately, Michigan had just started an honors program, and I was encouraged to join. To my chagrin classes were small and essays were required. I managed to thread a painful course through this minefield for two years, but the time was coming when I was to be judged solely on my non-existent writing skills. . . . Ironically, it was the competitive Johns Hopkins School of Medicine that came to my rescue. . . . To this day, among a backdrop of students who were universally able and mature, I am not sure whether or not they knew that I could not spell, punctuate, or produce even half-literate compositions.[10]

Clearly, Wyatt was destined to have a brilliant career as a research scientist and America's psychiatrist in chief. He wasted no time to become an employee-agent of the U.S. government:

I made my way to the National Institutes of Health, where I have had the great fortune to spend my professional career. I have always thought that one of our chief goals at the NIH is to take on challenges that others, hemmed in by grant requirements and promotion committees, cannot. The NIH is also the best place in the world for those of us who have never given up Tinker Toys. During my career I have focused on schizophrenia, which—though little understood—continues to cause untold suffering lifelong. My investigation into the course and roots of schizophrenia led me into research on sleep and imaging, psychopharmacology, biochemistry, neuroplasticity, economics, and epidemiology. . . . The article "Neuroleptics and the natural course of schizophrenia" grew out of my search for evidence that early intervention [that is, coercion and drugging while the subject is still a minor and is totally helpless to resist such intrusion] can change the course of schizophrenia. . . . And even if chronicity cannot be lessened, can early intervention lower the risk of suicide, substance abuse, and other problems that develop early on in the disease?

Wyatt knew on which side his bread was buttered. Here he pushes the two defining buttons of the therapeutic state: suicide and substance abuse.

He continues, "I believe that early intervention will almost certainly convey sufficient benefit in these latter areas to force a change in public health practices. . . . Throughout my career I have never expected to understand schizophrenia." Wisely, Wyatt made no attempt to understand the persons he dehumanized as "having schizophrenia."

On January 12, 1978, Wyatt and three other "researchers" published a paper in the *New England Journal of Medicine,* titled "Are Paranoid Schizophrenics Biologically Different from Other Schizophrenics?" Their answer was yes. They claimed to have demonstrated that the blood platelets of chronic nonparanoid schizophrenics exhibited a significantly lower level of monoamine oxidase (MAO) activity than did the platelets of chronic paranoid schizophrenics or normal controls. *In the same month,* Wyatt and four other "researchers" published a paper in the *American Journal of Psychiatry,* titled "Platelet Monoamine Oxidase in Chronic Schizophrenic Patients."[11] Their conclusion was that "there were no significant differences between the mean platelet MAO activities of 21 chronic paranoid schizophrenic patients compared with 18 chronic undifferentiated schizophrenic patients." What makes these two articles uniquely relevant is that both were coauthored by Dennis L. Murphy, chief of the Clinical Neuropharmacology Branch of the National Institute of Mental Health in Bethesda, Maryland, and Richard J. Wyatt, then chief of the Laboratory of Clinical Psychopharmacology at St. Elizabeth's Hospital in Washington, D.C.

The contradiction between these two reports created a tempest in a psychiatric teaspoon. On May 18, 1978, the *New England Journal of Medicine* published a series of letters, as well as a scathing editorial note, concerning the affair. In the lead letter, a psychiatrist noted the contradiction between the two articles cited and concluded, "It seems worthwhile to clarify how the same authors can come to such diametrically opposed conclusions—a clarification that I have been unable to extract from either article." In their reply, the authors "explained" that "we could not previously address ourselves to the then unpublished study by Berger et al. because it has been our policy not to discuss unpublished data in a published paper."[12] The editors of the *New England Journal of Medicine* were not satisfied:

We are as puzzled as Dr. Pager [the author of the letter] by the virtually simultaneous publication of two apparently contradictory papers, one in the *Journal* and the other in the *American Journal of Psychiatry*. Despite the fact that these papers share two coauthors in common, neither manuscript, as submitted, referred to the existence of the other. . . . We cannot be satisfied with the explanation given of this bizarre event. . . . To dismiss one's own discrepant results as being "unpublished data" and therefore not open to comment defies common sense and is, to say the least, disingenuous.[13]

Viewed in the context of psychiatry in which mendacity is the rule, rather than in the context of science in which mendacity is the exception, Wyatt's reporting in one paper that there is a significant difference in the platelet monoamine oxidase activities of paranoid schizophrenics and in another paper, published in the same month, that there is no such difference is not bizarre. The everyday cannot be deemed "bizarre"; not even the absurd belief that the biochemical properties of blood platelets are related to the etiology of the portmanteau human condition psychiatrists call "schizophrenia" can be deemed bizarre.

By psychiatric context, I refer to the moral arena in which defaming Leonardo da Vinci as a homosexual and Barry Goldwater as a schizophrenic is accepted as sophisticated medical diagnoses and where, as I show in this book, deceit and prevarication are the currency of everyday "professional" discourse. Such conduct, practiced consistently over many generations, inexorably affects every aspect of psychiatry, from the deceptive manipulation of the mental patient in the name of treatment to the deceptive manipulation of research in the name of science.

IV

Notwithstanding the similarities between authenticated forgeries as masterpieces and authenticated mental diseases as real diseases, there is a crucial difference between them. Art forgers never delude themselves about their work. Psychiatrists often do, often with tragic consequences. The murder of Wayne Fenton, a "renowned expert in the diagnosis and treatment of schizophrenia" and a high-ranking administrator at the National Institute of Mental Health, illustrates what happens when a "scientist" believes that schizophrenics have bad brains and ignores that they are persons who, like most people, prefer not to be incarcerated and forcibly drugged. On October 6, 2006, *Psychiatric News* reported:

> The murder of an NIMH administrator while trying to help a psychotic patient sent shockwaves through the mental health community. . . . [T]he potential nightmare in the life of a psychiatrist: a patient becomes violent, even homicidal, while the psychiatrist and the patient are alone in the psychiatrist's office. Wayne Fenton, M.D., often made remarks to this effect: "All anyone has to do is walk through any downtown area to appreciate that the lack of adequate treatment for patients with schizophrenia and other mental illnesses is a serious problem in this country. We wouldn't let our 80-year-old mother with Alzheimer's live on a [sewer] grate. Why is it all right for a 30-year-old daughter with schizophrenia?"[14]

The analogy is totally false and misleading. The management of incompetent persons—be they healthy babies or demented old people—is primarily a familial, economic, and legal matter. It is not, and ought not to be treated as, a "psychiatric problem." According to this construction, Fenton believed his self-serving analogy—that a strange man, presumed legally competent until proved to be legally incompetent, ought to be cared for like his own mother with Alzheimer's disease—and threatened a person *he* called "schizophrenic" with psychiatric incarceration and forced drugging. If it indeed happened—and the evidence points that way—then he had mainly himself to blame when his intended victim turned on him:

> Asked by a colleague to see a patient in crisis—who was reportedly suffering ongoing paranoid and complex delusions but *was now also noncompliant*—Fenton agreed. After all, Fenton was used to referrals of challenging patients. Even though it was Labor Day weekend, Fenton, director of the Division of Adult Translational Research and associate director for clinical affairs at NIMH, met with the 19-year-old patient and his father on Saturday, then made an appointment for follow-up the next week. However, on Sunday, according to court documents, the patient's father called Fenton, pleading with him to see his son again. *The patient reportedly was*

very agitated. He was unhappy with his medications and was refusing to take them, the father told Fenton. Holiday weekend or not, however, Fenton was known for his devotion to patients—especially those who were severely ill. *This patient was clearly seriously ill and needed help.*

That this man was "seriously ill and needed help" may have been apparent to Fenton and may be apparent to people who write for and read *Psychiatric News,* but it is not at all apparent to anyone with an ear for psychiatric lies. The "patient" did not ask Fenton for help. One of Fenton's colleagues and the "patient's" father asked for help. The "patient" beat Fenton to death and made no attempt to escape: "The patient, who remains in custody, was charged with first-degree murder. After pleading 'not criminally responsible' due to mental illness on September 18, he was awaiting transfer to a state psychiatric hospital where he will be evaluated to determine competency to stand trial."

At the beginning of his story, the reporter calls patient violence "the potential nightmare in the life of a psychiatrist." After describing what evidently happened, he flatly contradicts himself: "Wayne Fenton died while trying to help a seriously ill patient. Numerous colleagues contacted by *Psychiatric News* expressed profound shock at Fenton's death, yet many were not completely surprised. . . . APA President Pedro Ruiz, M.D., observed, 'We should not overreact and think that most patients with mental illness are more dangerous than the population at large. To do so would negate the work of Dr. Fenton with severely ill patients.'" The last three words are psychiatric code for individuals who, in the view of "correctly practicing" psychiatrists, ought to be locked up and drugged against their will. APA president Pedro Ruiz repeats the mandatory psychiatric mendacity that mental patients are no more dangerous than nonmental patients. This claim, too, the reporter himself contradicts:

Indeed, psychiatrists and mental health professionals are subject to a significantly higher risk of violent crime than most other categories of professionals. The U.S. Occupational Safety and Health Administration, the Bureau of Labor Statistics (BLS), and the Department of Justice (DoJ) agree that health care workers face some of the highest levels of job-related violence.

BLS statistics show that there were 69 homicides of health care personnel from 1996 through 2000. According to the DoJ's National Crime Victimization Survey for 1993 to 1999, the annual rate for nonfatal violent crime for all occupations was 12.6 per 1,000 workers. For physicians, the rate was 16.2, and for nurses it was 21.9. But for psychiatrists and mental health professionals, the rate was 68.2, and for mental health custodial workers, 69.

Trapped in their own lies, psychiatrists escalate them. Averting their eyes from the obvious connections between the practice of psychiatric coercion, especially incarceration, and the potential violence of the psychiatric prisoner, the experts demand more psychiatric power to coerce: "The circumstances surrounding Fenton's death 'speaks [sic] volumes about the extent to which the mental health system has unraveled,' said Mary Zdanowicz, executive director of the Treatment Advocacy Center. 'There really is no system left to respond when a person is having a psychiatric crisis. . . . It's so troubling to me that the knee-jerk reaction to this tragedy will be for people to say, "Most people with mental illness are not dangerous." But the fact of the matter is, some are.'"

Whether they talk about platelets or patients, diagnosis or treatment, law or liberty, psychiatrists remain stubbornly estranged from truth-telling. Their discourse typically begins with claims about mental illnesses being like other illnesses, proceeds to stories about the dangerousness of persons called "mental patients," and invariably ends with lamentations about the lack of adequate psychiatric services for this or that "population" and need for more government funding.

6 Lying

Pseudologist: liar. *Pseudologue:* pathological liar.
—*Webster's Third New International Dictionary*

In the seventeenth century, the malingerer wanted to be accepted as genuinely ill and avoided exposure. Today, the malingerer is automatically accepted as genuinely ill and seeks the limelight as a cured celebrity or "specially gifted researcher."

Psychiatrists never miss an opportunity to proclaim that "mental illness is like any other illness." This claim is supported by the medical profession, the political class, and the media. Not surprisingly, people regard psychiatrists as the foremost experts on mental illnesses. Psychologists, regularly confused with psychiatrists, often share that dubious distinction.

The expertise attributed to body doctors and soul doctors alike rests on their academic credentials and the licenses granted them by the states. In the United States, mental health professionals are often given extra credits if they have "suffered" and "recovered" from the mental illnesses they "research" and "treat." Laypersons, especially if they are socially or politically prominent, may also be credited with such special savvy. Examples abound.

Tipper Gore, wife of former vice president Albert Gore, is regarded as an expert on "clinical depression": "I suffered from depression and I underwent a very successful treatment. . . . Mental illness is a biochemical disorder. It happens in the brain, a physical part of the body."[1]

Betty Ford, wife of President Gerald Ford, went from alcoholic drug addict to expert on drug abuse, a "certification" Wikipedia describes as follows: "In 1978, the Ford family staged an intervention and forced her to confront her alcoholism and an addiction to opioid analgesics that had been prescribed in the early 1960s for a pinched nerve. 'I liked alcohol,' she wrote in her 1987 memoir. 'It made me feel warm. And I loved pills.' . . . In 1982, after her recovery, she established the Betty Ford Center in Rancho Mirage, California, for the treatment of chemical dependency."[2]

In other words, "madmen" and "madwomen" who commit psychiatric autos-da-fé—that is, who, after receiving the "services" of the psychiatric Inquisition, embrace coercive psychiatry as a miraculous force for "mental healing"—are model psychiatric educators and reformers. The classic case is that of Clifford Whittingham Beers (1876–1943).

A graduate of Yale University, Beers was socially well positioned to begin his appointed career as a financier. Evidently unenthusiastic about that prospect, he "tried" to kill himself. His failed suicide attempt was promptly attributed to manic depression, now called "bipolar disorder," and he was incarcerated for several years in several institutions, private and public. That experience helped him to "find himself," or, as he put it in his autobiography, *A Mind That Found Itself* (1908), helped his mind to do that job. Widely and favorably reviewed, his book became a best-seller, and is still in print. In 1909 Beers founded the National Commission for Mental Hygiene, and in 1913 he created the Clifford W. Beers Clinic in New Haven, the first outpatient mental health clinic in the United States. He remained a leader in the field until his retirement in 1939.[3] The Web site of the Clifford W. Beers Clinic describes his work as follows: "The personal odyssey of Clifford W. Beers can be likened to the mythical hero's journey to find himself. Through his journey, he brought new hope and inspiration into the world—and a national system of psychiatric treatment was eventually transformed. He is considered one of the founders of the mental health movement in America."[4]

Psychiatrists quickly recognized that Beers could be an asset to them and actively supported his efforts to legitimate "good" psychiatric coercion. Historians of psychiatry continue to venerate Beers as the founding father of American mental health reform, much as they view Benjamin Rush as the founding father of American psychiatry.

Today, perhaps the best-known psychiatric expert—whose credentials include having bipolar illness, a suicide attempt, treatment with lithium, as well as a professorship in psychiatry at the Johns Hopkins Medical School—is psychologist Kay Redfield Jamison (1946–). Although not a (medical) doctor, she "has been named one of the 'Best Doctors in the United States' and was chosen by *Time* magazine as a 'Hero of Medicine.' . . . Jamison is the recipient of the National Mental Health Association's William Styron Award (1995), the American Suicide Foundation Research Award (1996), the Community Mental Health Leadership Award (1999), and was a 2001 MacArthur Fellowship recipient."[5]

Jamison has written extensively about her alleged illness and near-death experience (NDE). On a Web site on NDE, under the heading "Dr. Kay Jamison's Near-Death Experience," we learn:

> Mental illness can trigger religious revelations and visions—even outof-body and near-death experiences. On this web page you will . . . read about one of the most distinguished scientists in the mental health field and her NDE which was triggered by a manic-depressive psychosis. Dr. Kay Jamison is the distinguished Professor of Psychiatry at the John Hopkins School of Medicine and co-author of the standard medical text taught there. Dr. Jamison is one of the foremost authorities on manic depressive illness. She is also a manic depressive herself. In her highly acclaimed book entitled *An Unquiet Mind,* Dr. Jamison describes a psychotic episode she had that transported her consciousness out of her body and into the solar system. . . . Jamison's consciousness traveled to Jupiter while she was enjoying the manic phase of her mental illness. The following is an excerpt from her excellent book and the account of her journey. "People go mad in idiosyncratic ways. Perhaps it was not surprising that, as a meteorologist's daughter, I found myself, in that glorious illusion of high summer days, gliding, flying, now and again lurching through cloud banks and ethers, past stars, and across fields of ice crystals. Even now, I can see in my mind's rather peculiar eye an extraordinary shattering and shifting of light; inconstant but ravishing colors laid out across miles of circling rings; and the almost imperceptible, somehow surprisingly pallid, moons of this Catherine wheel of a planet. I remember singing Fly Me to the Moon as I swept past those of Saturn, and thinking myself terribly funny. I saw and experienced that which had been only in dreams, or fitful fragments of aspiration. . . . Long after my psychosis cleared, and the medications took hold, it became part of what one remembers

forever, surrounded by an almost Proustian melancholy. Long since that extended voyage of my mind and soul, Saturn and its icy rings took on a elegiac beauty, and I don't see Saturn's image now without feeling an acute sadness at its being so far away from me, so unobtainable in so many ways."[6]

I

The name of psychologist and science writer Lauren Slater (1963–) belongs on this list of "mad persons" using their madness to build successful careers as celebrity experts on madness.

Slater's academic credentials are impeccable: a graduate of Brandeis University, she received a master's degree in psychology from Harvard University and a doctorate in psychology from Boston University. In 2000, when she was only thirty-seven years old, Slater published her autobiography, titled *Lying: A Metaphorical Memoir*:

> In *Lying* I have written a book in which in some cases I cannot and in other cases I will not say the facts. I am, after all, the grandchild of Kant, of Heisenberg. . . . All I know for sure is this. I have been ill much of my life. Illness has claimed much of my life. Illness has claimed my imagination, my brain, my body, and everything I do I see through its feverish scrim. All I can tell you is this. Illness, medicine itself, is the ultimate narrative; there is no truth there, as diagnoses come in and out of vogue as fast as yearly fashions.[7]

Slater's assertion, "Illness, medicine itself, is the ultimate narrative; there is no truth there," is false. She conceals it by equating medicine with diagnosis. However, medicine is concerned with diseases, not diagnoses. Only psychiatry is concerned with diagnoses, because in psychiatry diagnoses are diseases ("disorders").

Slater says her father was "a Hebrew school teacher," and her mother a professional liar, a "woman . . . [who] rarely spoke the truth. . . . From my mother I learned that truth is bendable, that what you wish is every bit as real as what you are."[8] Slater then relates the "narrative truth" of her life, more blessed than blighted by "illness":

I have epilepsy. Or I feel I have epilepsy. Or I wish I had epilepsy, so I could find a way of explaining the dirty, spastic glittering place in my mother's heart. Epilepsy is a fascinating disease because some epileptics are liars. . . . Doctors don't know why this is. . . . I don't know where this is my mother or where this is my illness, or whether, like her, I am just confusing fact with fiction, and there is no epilepsy, just a clenched metaphor, a way of telling you what I have to tell you: my tale.[9]

In short, Slater's credo is that there is no valid boundary between truth and lie, fact and fantasy, real disease and imagined disease. Her mocking prose style is an effective vehicle for her tale of deviousness. She writes, "Dear Reader: Every night before dinner I say grace. I light two white tapers, and even though I was born a Jew, I clasp my hands and give thanks to a Christian God for the kindness he has shown."[10] Slater has a husband and two children, but she pretends to be dining alone. She enlivens her memoir with touches of prurience and violence:

But I, Jewish by blood, have always preferred churches, because a seizure in a synagogue means disruption and embarrassment, whereas a seizure in a church is part of the holy atmosphere. Churches are places for the two-tongued and the fainters, for broken bodies. Christ himself had his body broken, his back snapped on the board of the cross, little nails driven right through his lifelines. He died up there, stinking and bloody, and tell me this: Where in a synagogue can you find such a sight, a synagogue all clean and quiet, smelling of bleach and law? . . . The sun died and was reborn again, in a flare of lemons. . . . Jesus held my hand, both of us were naked, and, I hate to admit it, aroused.[11]

In a chapter titled "Memo" to her publisher, Slater imitates Wittgenstein's style in the *Tractatus* (1921), listing one "point" after another: "1. This is a difficult book, I know. There was or was not a cherry tree. The seizures are real or something else. I am an epileptic or I have Munchausen's. . . . 3. . . . I, for one, am a slippery sort, but I believe I'm also an honest sort, because I admit my slipperiness. . . . 14. The neural mechanism that undergirds the lie is the same neural mechanism that helps us make narrative. . . . 17. My *memoir*, please. Sell it as nonfiction, please." This piece of überchutzpah reminds one of Mary McCarthy's famous quip about her fellow writer Lillian Hellman: "Every word she writes is a lie, including 'and' and 'the.'"[12]

Growing tired of her role as fake epileptic, Slater joins Alcoholics Anonymous (AA). Well, she doesn't *really* join the group. She wanders into an AA meeting and is embraced as one of their own by a man with "nice breath": "I didn't know how to explain what I was doing here, and I thought if he found out I wasn't an alcoholic, he'd get mad, and so I said, 'Well . . . seven months.'" And so begins a new chapter in *Slater's Travels*: "Most of the time my lie didn't bother me, because AA, like any disease, is about so much more that its symptoms. AA is about life, and honesty, God and desperation, and desire, and these things are relevant to anyone."[13] With considerable literary skill, Slater composes effective psychiatric propaganda by conflating diagnosis, disease, desire, desperation, AA, and God:

> Alcoholism and epilepsy, so many vector points. Both can come back anytime. Even more important, both are more than just physical diseases. Both are personality problems as well. AAers describe addiction as an allergy of the body coupled with an obsession of the mind and an impoverishment of the spirit. For me, epilepsy, along with what doctors called my temporal lobe epileptic personality disorder, was also a psychological, spiritual, and physical thing. . . . Let me tell you, I fit right in. "We drink," the AAers said, "because there is a hole in our souls," a hole they had tried to fill with many marvelous liquors, as I had tried to fill with intoxicants of tall tales, the intoxicant of attention lavished on the patient and the poet, me.[14]

Slater beats the reader to the punch: she confesses to being an inveterate liar, unmasking herself before anyone else could do so. Notwithstanding such evidence, Slater takes herself seriously as a science writer and is taken seriously by publishers, psychologists, psychiatrists, journalists, and probably many readers. She has contributed to the *New York Times*, *Harper's*, and *Elle*, and has won several literary awards. Wikipedia describes her as "a freelance writer specializing in psychology, mental illness, and women's health," noting that the *Village Voice* has called her "the closest thing we have to a doyenne of psychiatric disorder."

II

Slater's first book, *Welcome to My Country: A Therapist's Memoir of Madness* (1997), established her reputation as a talented writer. *Publishers Weekly* praised Slater's "empathy with her patients . . . tempered by her own bout of treated mental disability. . . . [T]he author ponders anew the mystery of why she 'managed somehow to leave behind at least for now what looks like wreckage, and shape something solid from life,' while others have not. This debut book opens a vista on emotional and mental distress." The reviewer must have accepted the author's claim that the story she relates is true. Yet neither here—nor in her "metaphorical memoir," published four years later—does Slater cite any behavior that would have justified or required psychiatrists to incarcerate her. She was happy to be a voluntary mental patient, in or out of hospitals. The reviewer for the *Library Journal*, too, had only praise for "this fittingly subtitled work. Slater introduces the schizophrenic, depressed, and suicidal patients she treats. Painting tender portraits of these troubled souls . . . Slater's personal struggle with mental illness is touchingly revealed when she journeys to the treatment facility wherein she lived for long periods in order to treat a patient with problems reminiscent of her own."[15]

In 2004, three years after causing a sensation with *Lying*, Slater escalated the controversy swirling around her persona by publishing an ostensibly serious piece of writing, titled *Opening Skinner's Box: Great Psychological Experiments of the Twentieth Century*. The book opens with this sentence: "I did my first psychological experiment when I was fourteen years old."[16] For the next two and a half pages, Slater says nothing about her ostensible subject; instead, she tells us about her favorite subject, herself.

Professionals who call their work "experiments" are empiricists, that is, they offer repeatable, objective evidence for their factual claims. But Slater, as we have seen, dislikes facts. She prefers fabrications that are *truer* than facts: "We most fully integrate that which is told as a tale. My hope is that some of these experiments will be more fully taken in by readers *now that they have been translated into narrative form*."[17] The proper person to do the translating is, of course, Slater.

Opening Skinner's Box is an ambitious attempt to revision the works of other psychologists as "stories": "Our lives, after all, are not data points and means and modes; they are stories—absorbed, reconfigured, rewritten. We most fully integrate that which is told as a tale. . . . Can we even define as disease syndromes that have no clear-cut physiological etiology or pathophysiology? Is psychology, which deals half in metaphor, half in statistics, really a science at all? Isn't science itself a form of metaphor?"[18] Here and elsewhere, Slater toys with the idea that mental illness is a metaphor and that psychiatry is, in toto, a big lie. But, eager to pose as a loyal mental health professional and sophisticated critic, she avoids that temptation, if it is one.

Slater devotes one chapter of *Opening Skinner's Box* to Rosenhan's so-called pseudopatient study and to her attempt to "replicate" it. She sets the stage for her account by revealing that she is not merely a liar but also a sadist: "He lost his wife. He lost his daughter. He lost his mind to a series of small strokes and now David Rosenhan, Stanford professor emeritus of law and psychology, now he can barely breathe." She sprinkles the rest of her chapter on Rosenhan with unflattering remarks about him, such as the following: "Rosenhan was a boxy man in his thirties when all this happened. He was known as an entertainer, holding at his home seders for as many as fifty people. . . . Says good friend and Stanford colleague Florence Keller, 'David's the only man I know who enlarged his house *after* his kids left for college, so he could have more revelers over.' Then Keller pauses. 'He had a way with words,' she says. 'But you also never felt you really knew him. He had a mask on.' Indeed he did."[19]

Slater's passion for what she calls "stories" leads her to misstating elementary facts, such as the historical context into which she places the Rosenhan study: "It was 1972. Spiro Agnew had just resigned. Thomas Szaz [*sic*] had written *The Myth of Mental Illness*."[20] The book was written in the mid- to late 1950s and published in 1961. She calls R. D. Laing "Lang." Numerous reviewers noted these misspellings and attributed them to sloppiness. Is that right? Or might they be Slater's sly way of hinting that her narrative is *hers* and has little to do with what she claims to be describing? If her acknowledgments are true, approximately a dozen persons have read all or parts of her manuscript, yet none noted these glaring errors of fact.

III

Slater's alleged re-creation of the Rosenhan experiment makes it clear that she is writing fiction, albeit she and her publisher (W. W. Norton) pretend that she is presenting popularized science. Although she has no idea of "the actual day that Rosenhan departed for one of Pennsylvania's state hospitals," she writes, "The actual day that Rosenhan departed for one of Pennsylvania's state hospitals was brilliant. The sky was a frosty pre-winter blue, the trees like brushes dipped in pots of paint, turned upward and wet with color."[21] The rest of her account is fabrication and fantasy, anchored to a few facts. The reader has no way to know what part, if any, is true. Slater's description of her plan to repeat Rosenhan's hoax confirms the impression that she prefers storytelling to truth-telling:

> Many things are the same. The sky is poignant blue. The trees are turning. . . . In the stores there will soon be plastic pumpkins. . . . My own child is too young for pumpkins; she has just turned two, and perhaps *because of Rosenhan and all the research he has spawned into "etiology and pathogenesis," I often worry about her brain, which I picture pink-red and rumpled in its casement.*
>
> "You are WHAT?" my husband says to me.
>
> "I'm going to try it," I say. "Repeat the experiment exactly as Rosenhan and his confederates did it and see if I get admitted." . . .
>
> "I'm coming too," he finally says.
>
> No. He is not. Someone has to watch the baby. I do my preparations. I don't shower or *shave* [*sic*] for five days.[22]

As sick humor, it works quite well, but it quickly gets tiresome. As in *Lying,* Slater toys with the reader and displays a lack of moral seriousness about her religious identity. She is in the hospital emergency room being interviewed by a nurse: "'Race,' she says. 'Jewish,' I say. I wonder if I should have said Protestant. The fact is I am Jewish, but I'm also paranoid. . . . I don't want the Jewish thing used against me."[23]

Slater knows that she is lying and lets us know it, too. Commitment policies are a matter of law, not science. Like the speed limit on highways, they change from time to time. During the thirty years since Rosenhan's study, the policy of maximum institutionalization has been replaced by the policy of maximum non- and deinstitutionalization.[24] "Of what am I so scared? No one can commit me. Since Rosenhan's study . . . commitment laws are far more stringent, and so long as I deny homicidal or suicidal urges, I'm a free woman. 'You're a free woman, Lauren,' I tell myself, while in the back of my mind is that rushing hysterical river with its buried alluvium and stink—smash smash."[25]

Slater's psychiatric critics, as I shall show presently, make a mistake in taking her seriously, examining *Opening Skinner's Box* as if its subject had something to do with its title. Slater has no real interest in, or understanding of, Rosenhan's hoax or any of the other matters that are the ostensible subjects of her book. These are merely hooks on which she hangs her pseudo-autobiographical masturbation about *her* "hysterical river" and "buried alluvium" and other metaphors that refer to nothing but her own supremely interesting "mind":

> It's a little fun, going into ERs and playing this game, so over the next eight days I do it eight more times, nearly the number of admissions Rosenhan arranged. Each time, of course, I am *denied* admission—I deny that I am a threat and I assure people I am able to do my work and take care of my child—but strangely enough, most times I am given a diagnosis of depression with psychotic features, even though, I am now sure, after a thorough self-inventory and the solicited opinions of my friends and my physician brother, I am really not depressed. . . . I am prescribed a total of twenty-five antipsychotics and sixty antidepressants. . . . Later on, I fill my prescriptions at the all-night pharmacy. And then, in the spirit of experimentation, I take the antipsychotic Risperdal, just one pill, and I fall into such a deep charcoal sleep that not a sound comes through, and I float, weightless, in another world, seeing vague shapes—trees, rabbits, angels, ships—but as hard as I peer, I can only wonder what is what.[26]

Readers who believe any of this fantasizinig have only themselves to blame. Slater, as we saw, opens her chapter on Rosenhan by pitilessly depicting him as a ruined man. She ends it by pretending to pity him:

I'd like very much to help Rosenhan, who as of this writing is still in a West Coast hospital, paralyzed, even his vocal cords. His friend Florence Keller says to me, "He's had so many tragedies. . . . It's been too much for him." Therefore I'd like to tell him I redid his study and had a grand old time, because I think it would please him to know this. He is, now, at seventy-nine years old, at the eve of his life and will soon perform the greatest experiment of all, the stepping over into another world, from where the results are never returned. . . . I don't even know the man, but I have an unreasonable fondness for him. I am partial to jokesters, to adventurers, to people in pain. As an ex-mental patient . . . [27]

IV

Opening Skinner's Box precipitated a battle between Slater and her psychiatric critics. In April 2006, Mark Moran, who writes regularly for *Psychiatric News,* presented a detailed account of it:

Psychiatrists and a popular science writer have collided over claims made in a recently published book that revives the controversy about a 30-year-old study questioning the validity of psychiatric diagnoses. . . . Robert Spitzer, M.D., of Columbia University College of Physicians and Surgeons, and other psychiatrists and psychologists have called into question claims made by science writer Lauren Slater in her 2004 book, *Opening Skinner's Box: Great Psychological Experiments of the 20th Century.* . . . Slater also reported the results of her own exercise in posing as a patient. . . . "When I read it, it just didn't make sense," [Spitzer] told *Psychiatric News.* . . . Spitzer, who was editor of *DSM-III* and has been an important figure in the evolution and refinement of psychiatric diagnoses, said he requested to see evidence of Slater's experiment—including files from her visits to the ERs or names of psychiatrists or hospitals—but that she has not produced them. And he told *Psychiatric News* he is highly skeptical about the medications Slater reported she was prescribed. . . . Others are less circumspect. "I believe the data were fabricated," psychiatrist Mark Zimmerman, M.D., told *Psychiatric News.* "As a researcher, I know that if anyone has a question about my data, how easy it is to produce data files, and Slater hasn't done that."[28]

Spitzer was no match for Slater's chutzpah. In the November 2005 issue of the *Journal of Nervous and Mental Disorders,* Slater explained that her book is not a "study" and cannot be critiqued as such:

> The book features not only the experiments and the experimenters, but me, as well, and my husband, and my daughter and my pet raccoon. In any case, such a colorful cast of characters and deeply personal details . . . are in and of themselves enough to make abundantly obvious to any and all readers that we are not here dealing with an academic inquiry, or "study." That Spitzer et al. have chosen to label my work as a study is a silly and troubling mischaracterization. . . . The authors also fully understand that my use of the word "experiment" is of course vernacular, as in, "honey, let's experiment with this recipe tonight." It would be far more useful, and appropriate, if the authors would drop the bloated and obfuscatory remarks, hunched and hiding as they are behind the veneer of "science," and claim their point in plain language. Their point, as far as I can see, is that they think I lied, which probably would not bother them so much if my alleged "lie" did not result in narcissistic injury.

Psychiatrists lie with the vocabulary of psychiatric diagnoses, prognoses, and treatments, and believe their lies are truths. Slater lies with fabrications couched in psychiatric jargon. Whether she lies to herself as well, she doesn't tell us.

With Slater's impostures our story comes full circle, from poor Parisian girls lying for room and board and a little attention to a professional psychologist lying for fame and royalties.

Tacitly, psychiatrists have always known that their subject was lies, but concealed the sordid ordinariness of this truism by attaching a host of impressive medical-sounding terms to them, hinting at extraordinarily complicated and interesting diseases. One such label was "pseudologia fantastica," which is not currently in the *Diagnostic and Statistical Manual of Mental Disorders,* but remains widely used: "Pseudologia fantastica is one of several terms applied by psychiatrists to the behavior of habitual or compulsive lying. It was first described in the medical literature in 1891. . . . Pseudologia fantastica is part of a spectrum of factious disorders, and may be associated with Munchausen syndrome, imposture, and peregrination. . . .

Other related terms are 'factitious disorder,' Mythomania and 'Munchausen syndrome.'"[29]

Since all deceptions share some common features, "Slater syndrome" may be said to be a type of pseudologia fantastica or "résumé fraud," that is, cheating to get a good job or, having one, to inflate one's achievements in academe, the job market, the military, and so on.[30]

V

I have tried to show that professionals in the mental health field are, *au fond,* impostors, pretending to have expertise they cannot possess. Being an expert about mental illnesses is like being an expert about ghosts or unicorns. Not surprisingly, some or many mental health experts come to feel like impostors, like frauds. This self-perception or self-assessment conflicts, however, with the perception and assessment of their peers and superiors. What are the impostors to do? They "diagnose" their "condition" the Impostor Syndrome, which Wikipedia describes as follows: "The Impostor Syndrome, or Impostor Phenomenon, sometimes called Fraud Syndrome, is not an officially recognized psychological disorder, but has been the subject of a number of books and articles by psychologists and educators. Individuals experiencing this syndrome seem unable to internalize their accomplishments. Regardless of what level of success they may have achieved in their chosen field of work or study . . . they remain convinced internally that they do not deserve the success they have achieved and are really frauds."[31]

The leading expert on the Impostor Syndrome is Valerie Young, "a trim, businesslike woman who calls herself a 'recovering impostor.' After learning about the syndrome in graduate school—and identifying strongly with it— she left academe with a Ph.D. in education and hit the lecture circuit. She has delivered her talk, 'How to Feel as Bright and Capable as Everyone Seems to Think You Are,' at dozens of campuses."[32]

In the mental health professions, there are no frauds; there can be no frauds. Why? Because the frauds are not impostors but mentally ill mental health experts who temporarily lack insight into their illness. When they recover and regain their insight, they realize—as Valerie Young did—that they are competent and compassionate "therapists" who treat life-threatening diseases and save "seriously mentally ill" patients from horrors worse than self-determined death (suicide). The cure for the Impostor Syndrome is to become a self-confident impostor.

Acting—pretending to be someone one is not—is what actors do. So-called mentally ill persons—who pretend to be disabled by illnesses that do not exist—do the same thing. When the imposture is performed onstage, the audience interprets it as humorous. When the imposture is performed in a "clinical setting," the audience is expected to suspend its critical faculties and accept the impersonation at face value, with compassion for the "suffering victim" and reverence toward the impostor.

Religious miracles and mental illnesses resemble one another. Each forms the foundational lies of a grand system of beliefs and social practices. Ridiculing such false beliefs undermines important social values. Religion thus banishes laughter from the church; medicine banishes laughter from the clinic. Charcot's clinical theater was a watermark. The public was permitted to laugh at the hysterics' performances. Doctors were expected to take them seriously as the signs of neurological diseases. Slater's literary performance is a quasi-medical comedy, misinterpreted as medical autobiography and psychological research. Wittingly or not, *Lying* is a tour de force of Wildean "Bunburyism."

Bunbury is a fictional character, the creation of Algernon Moncrieff, the protagonist in Oscar Wilde's (1854–1900) great comedy of manners, *The Importance of Being Earnest* (1895). Algernon, an aristocratic young Londoner, pretends to have a friend named Bunbury who lives in the country and is frequently in ill health. Whenever he wants to avoid an unwelcome social obligation, he justifies absenting himself by having to visit his "sick friend." Calling this practice "Bunburying," Wilde introduces the term—now a part of the English language—in the following dialogue:

ALGERNON [speaking to his best friend, Jack/Ernest Worthing]. I suspected that, my dear fellow! I have Bunburyed all over Shropshire on two separate occasions. Now, go on. Why are you Ernest in town and Jack in the country? . . . Literary criticism is not your forte, my dear fellow. Don't try it. . . . What you really are is a Bunburyist. I was quite right in saying you were a Bunburyist. You are one of the most advanced Bunburyists I know.

JACK. What on earth do you mean?

ALGERNON. You have invented a very useful younger brother called Ernest, in order that you may be able to come up to town as often as you like. I have invented an invaluable permanent invalid called Bunbury, in order that I may be able to go down into the country whenever I choose. Bunbury is perfectly invaluable. If it wasn't for Bunbury's extraordinary bad health, for instance, I wouldn't be able to dine with you at Willis's to-night.[33]

Laughing at sacred cows and cultural taboos is, however, no laughing matter, as Wilde and many others have discovered. The proverb says, "He who laughs last, laughs best." This statement is patently untrue if the authorities possess the power to punish the mocker and the zeal to use it.

Epilogue

The Burden of Responsibility

Responsibility: A detachable burden easily shifted to the shoulders of
God, Fate, Fortune, Luck or one's neighbor. In the days of astrology it
was customary to unload it upon a star.

—Ambrose Bierce (1842–1914?), *The Unabridged
Devil's Dictionary*

Human beings are choice-making animals. The freedom to make choices
is both a blessing and a curse. Depending on age, temperament, information, and alternatives, some people experience the opportunity for choice as
exhilarating, others as tormenting. Traditionally, it was one of the functions
of religion to relieve people of choices. Today, psychiatry—pharmacracy and
the therapeutic state—performs the same job.

Karl Jaspers understood this point very well. But, writing almost one
hundred years ago, he identified only the part the patient played in the
drama: "Generally formulated, we may say that these people ["neurotics"]
are *determined that events for which they are accountable and in which they are
understandably concerned shall be taken as mere happenings, for which they are
entirely irresponsible.*"[1] The psychiatric profession was happy to oblige.

Life is an unending series of choices and, therefore, "problems in living."
Ordinary choices—such as what to have for breakfast—we ignore as trivial.
Extraordinary choices—such as whether to kill ourselves—we dismiss as the
symptoms of mental illness. The profession of psychiatry rests on, and caters
to, the ubiquitous human desire to avoid and evade, indeed deny the very possibility of, morally "unthinkable" choices. We use the rhetoric of psychiatry to
transform such choices into medical-technical problems and "solve" them by

112

appropriate "medical treatments." This discourse is why deception is intrinsic to the principles of psychiatry, and coercion-as-cure to its practices.

We cannot imagine life in a society bereft of psychiatry. For a long time, people could not imagine life in a society without gods and slaves. However, there came a time when, in some parts of the world, the despotisms of religion and slaveholding were abolished.

It is possible that religious, political, psychiatric, or some other kinds of evasions of personal responsibility will always be necessary for our existence as social beings. It is also possible that, in the future, some people, somewhere, will become as passionately interested in the pursuit of personal responsibility as they have been, for the past several centuries in the West, in the pursuit of personal liberty. When and if that time comes, the psychiatric enterprise will disappear and become of historical interest only.

I

The struggle against what Nietzsche called the "*pia fraus* [holy lie]" of the "improvers of mankind" remains the same through the ages, only the identity of the "improvers" changes.[2] This consideration led me to compare Lord Acton's reflections on the subversion of responsibility by the Roman Catholic Church and my reflections on Organized Psychiatry performing that role today.

John Emerich Edward Dalberg Acton (1834–1902), known usually as Lord Acton, descendant of an old, wealthy Roman Catholic family, was educated in England, Scotland, and Germany. He tried to, but as a Catholic could not, gain admission to Cambridge. Educated privately, he became a pupil of Johann Joseph Ignaz von Döllinger (1799–1890), the famous German theologian, Catholic priest, and church historian. Acton was master of the principal foreign languages and was personally acquainted with many of the great historians and politicians of his day.

In politics, Acton was a classical liberal, an opponent of power concentrated in a single source. He considered the federal structure of the United States a perfect guarantor of individual liberties and, during the Civil War, supported the Confederacy for its defense of states' rights against a centralizing government. In 1859, Acton settled in England, entered for a brief period the House of Commons, and in 1869 was raised to the peerage by Queen Victoria.

In 1870, under the influence of Pope Pius IX, the Vatican declared the dogma of papal infallibility. This kind of concentration of power was anathema to Acton. He became alienated, but never seceded, from the church. It saddened him, also, that his views regarding the Vatican led him to become alienated from his great teacher and friend, Döllinger. It was in the context of this conflict that, in 1887, in a letter to Bishop Mandell Creighton (1843–1901), Acton made his famous pronouncement: "I cannot accept your canon that we are to judge Pope and King unlike other men, with a favorable presumption that they did no wrong. If there is any presumption it is the other way against the holders of power, increasing as the power increases. Historic responsibility has to make up for want of legal responsibility. Power tends to corrupt and absolute power corrupts absolutely."[3]

Today, most people who quote Lord Acton's "dictum" are unaware that it refers to papal power and was made by a Catholic. In 1882, Acton, by this time alienated from Döllinger, writes him, "I came, very slowly and reluctantly indeed to the conclusion that [the great Catholic notabilities] were dishonest. And I found out a special reason for their dishonesty in the desire to keep up the credit of authority in the Church. . . . When I got to understand history from the sources, especially from unpublished sources, the reason of all this became obvious. There was a conspiracy to deceive. . . . That men might believe the Pope it was resolved to make them believe that vice is virtue and falsehood truth."[4]

It requires no ill will toward the Church of Psychiatry to see the striking parallels between Acton's critique of Vatican-sponsored mendacity and my critique of APA-sponsored mendacity. Acton regarded the claim of papal infallibility as evidence of intolerable religious arrogance and power. I regard psychiatric infallibility—the unfalsifiability and irrefutability of psychiatric diagnoses backed by mental health laws—as evidence of intolerable psychiatric arrogance and power. Acton continues:

> It cannot be faith in the true sense, which a man defends by immoral means. . . . [B]elief is not sincere when the believer is not sincere. . . . Therefore men who were outwardly defenders of religion appeared to me

in reality advocates of deceit and murder. . . . They preached falsehood and murder. . . . Seeing this wickedness in the present, in men apparently excellent, I cannot doubt its existence in the past. And therefore I am very unwilling, in morals, and in discussing great men, to make allowances for their time. I allow for what they could not know. I do not allow for what they might have known. I insist upon the greater guilt of greater men. . . . Just as the people of the Commune seem to me altogether odious, so do the people of the Vatican. . . . I have never found that people go wrong from ignorance, but from want of consciousness. Even the ignorant are ignorant because they wish to be—ignorant in bad faith.[5]

In a melancholy tone, Acton concludes: "I find that I am alone. . . . I cannot obey any conscience but my own."[6] Commenting on Acton's conflict with the church, Damien McElrath and James Holland, the editors of *Lord Acton: The Decisive Decade,* point out what ought to be obvious but is not:

When, in 1870, the Vatican declared the doctrine of Papal Infallibility, Acton "thought he witnessed the triumph of error in history." Indeed, he had. But Acton—passionate equally about truth and religion, liberty and responsibility—seemed not to have grasped that *factual error validated as Doctrinal Truth is essential for the survival of organizations whose aim is to satisfy man's unquenchable thirst to be relieved of the burden of moral responsibility.* Acton was unafraid of truth and responsibility. Indeed, he was eager to seek them regardless of cost, hence his nobly tragic struggle to reconcile Veracity with Religion, in particular Catholicism. . . . The result was Acton's inclination to the belief that the doctrine's supporters were guilty of something more than ignorance. One need only count the recurrence of the word "Lüge" (lie) or other words of similar meaning in his letters to Döllinger during the Council to realize that the ghost of Catholic mendacity, which was to stalk him for next two decades, assumes its amorphous shape at this time.[7]

II

Although the church diluted the concept of responsibility here on earth, it extended its reach and increased its severity in the hereafter. Psychiatry went much further: it abolished the concept of responsibility and, with it, the concepts of guilt and innocence, and replaced punishment with the irrefutable and ineradicable stigmata of psychiatric "diagnoses" and "treatments." "Modern psychiatry," I wrote in 1970, "dehumanize[s] man by denying . . . the existence, or even the possibility, of personal responsibility, central to the concept of man as moral agent."[8] It accomplishes that evil by treating responsibility, following Ambrose Bierce, as "a detachable burden easily shifted to the shoulders of God, Fate, Fortune, Luck or one's neighbor. In the days of astrology it was customary to unload it upon a star." In our day, it is not merely customary but, in matters that really count, even mandatory to unload personal responsibility on mental illness ("He snapped, had a breakdown, battled his demons, was on drugs, went off prescribed medication," and so forth).

Moreover, in Acton's day, the separation of church and state was a familiar idea and an established political practice in many countries. Hence, the church's power and moral failures affected only persons who chose to be its adherents (and their children). Our predicament, if such it be, is more serious. We live at a time when the alliance of psychiatry and the state is generally taken for granted as an *unalterable social fact* and *unquestionable moral good*. Everyone, regardless of personal choice, is affected, directly or indirectly, by the powers of the therapeutic state.

Given its limited legal-political powers at the time, Acton's church did not try to purge the world of its critics, much less intimidate them into becoming its crypto-supporters. In contrast, in our day, the alliance of psychiatry and the state has enabled pharmacracy to do that very thing. Its so-called critics—who call themselves "antipsychiatrists," "critical psychiatrists," "ethical psychiatrists," "postpsychiatrists," "ex-mental patients," "voice hearers," and so on—oppose one or another psychiatric "diagnosis" or "treatment," sometimes even psychiatric coercion. But they draw back from defending an ethic based on nonviolence, personal responsibility for public actions (as distinct from private actions, called "thoughts"), and every person's inalienable right to *his or her* life and death—lest they appear uncompassionate and, perish the thought, unscientific and illiberal (in the modern, statist sense of "liberal"). Thus, they endorse—explicitly or by the assent of silence—psychiatry's war on personal responsibility, epitomized by the wars on drugs, mental illness, and suicide and by the insanity defense in its various incarnations.

"Truth," said Thomas Jefferson (1743–1826), "will do well enough if left to shift for herself. She seldom has received much aid from the power of great men to whom she is rarely known and seldom welcome. She has no need of force to procure entrance into the minds of men. . . . It is error alone which needs the support of government."[9] Jefferson was right in applying this principle to religion: modern states should not (and for the most part do not) lend their coercive powers to the support of the clerical lies of priests. Nor should they lend their coercive powers to the support of the clinical lies of psychiatrists. As long as that is not the case, serious persons ought not to take psychiatry seriously—except as a threat to reason, responsibility, and liberty.

Notes
Bibliography
Index

Notes

Abbreviation

SE   *The Standard Edition of the Complete Psychological Works of Sigmund Freud.* 24 vols. London: Hogarth Press, 1953–1974.

Preface

1. "Thomas Carlyle (1795–1881)," http://www.bartleby.com/100/387.html.
2. Thomas Szasz, *Heresies,* 113, slightly modified. In *Heresies* I called the art and science of lying "mendacitology," a Greco-Latin neologism. The *Oxford English Dictionary* defines *pseudology* as "speaking falsely" and dates its use to the sixteenth century.

Introduction: The Invention of Psychopathology

1. Thomas Szasz, "Malingering: 'Diagnosis' or Social Condemnation?"
2. See Thomas Szasz, *Insanity: The Idea and Its Consequences,* 174–81.
3. See Associated Press, "Duke Lacrosse Players File Lawsuit," *New York Times,* Oct. 5, 2007, http://www.nytimes.com/aponline/us/AP-DukeLacrosse.html?hp; Associated Press, "Duke Prosecutor Sentenced to Day in Jail," Sept. 2, 2007, http://www.usatoday.com/news/nation/2007-08-31-nifong-jail_N.htm.
4. See Thomas Szasz, *Law, Liberty, and Psychiatry: An Inquiry into the Social Uses of Mental Health Practices.*
5. See Szasz, *Insanity;* and Szasz, *Liberation by Oppression: A Comparative Study of Slavery and Psychiatry.*
6. There are subtle but important differences among the performances these terms denote. A forged masterpiece is an original work by a forger, not a copy of the imitated artist's work: it is falsely attributed to the imitated artist. A counterfeit product is a copy of a real product, as exact a facsimile as the counterfeiter is capable of producing: it is not, in any sense, an original creation of the "counterfeiter." The forger and counterfeiter credit others

for their own work. The plagiarist credits himself for the work of another. All seek to profit by deception.

7. L. MacFarquhar, "Bag Man: Cracking Down on Fashion Fakes," 129. See also M. Fackler, "Fearing Crime, Japanese Wear the Hiding Place," *New York Times,* Oct. 20, 2007, http://www.nytimes/com/2007/10/20/world/asia/20japan.html?hp; and T. Hafner, "Tiffany and eBay in Fight over Fakes," *New York Times,* Nov. 27, 2007, http://www.nytimes .com/2007/11/27/technology/27ebay.html?ref=todayspaper.

8. M. S. Micale, "Hysteria and Its Historiography: The Future Perspective," 80 (emphasis added).

9. Emanuel Rubin and John L. Farber, *Pathology,* 2; Alvan R. Feinstein, *Clinical Judgment,* 119–21; David M. Reese, "Fundamentals: Rudolf Virchow and Modern Medicine," 105–8; René Leriche quoted in G. Canguilhem, *On the Normal and the Pathological,* 46.

10. Erwin H. Ackerknecht, *Rudolf Virchow: Doctor, Statesman, Anthropologist,* v.

11. Thomas Szasz, *The Myth of Mental Illness: Foundations of a Theory of Personal Conduct.*

12. E. Kinetz, "Is Hysteria Real? Brain Images Say Yes," *New York Times,* Sept. 26, 2006, http://www.nytimes.com/2006/09/26/science/26hysteria.html?ex=1159848000& en=08644dbf03819ba6&ei=5070&emc=eta1.

13. Thomas Szasz, *Fatal Freedom: The Ethics and Politics of Suicide*; Szasz, *Pharmacracy: Medicine and Politics in America*; Szasz, *The Medicalization of Everyday Life: Selected Essays.*

14. Thomas Szasz, "Bootlegging Humanistic Values Through Psychiatry"; "Assisted Suicide Is Bootleg Suicide," *Los Angeles Times,* Nov. 23, 2001.

15. Paul Lerner, *Hysterical Men: War, Psychiatry, and the Politics of Trauma in Germany, 1890–1930,* 7 (emphasis added).

16. Szasz, *Pharmacracy.*

17. Jonas Robitscher, *The Powers of Psychiatry,* 35–36.

18. See Thomas Szasz, *The Manufacture of Madness: A Comparative Study of the Inquisition and the Mental Health Movement.*

19. Richard von Krafft-Ebing, *Psychopathia Sexualis, with Special Reference to the Antipathic Sexual Instinct: A Medico-Forensic Study,* vi–vii, 52–54.

20. Richard P. Feynman and R. Leighton, *What Do You Care What Other People Think? Further Adventures of a Curious Character,* 14.

21. R. Kennedy, "If the Copy Is an Artwork, Then What's the Original?" *New York Times,* Dec. 6, 2007, http://www.nytimes.com/2007/12/06/arts/design/06prin.html.

22. Ernst von Feuchtersleben, *The Principles of Medical Psychology, Being the Outline of a Course of Lectures,* 74–75.

23. Thomas Szasz, *Ceremonial Chemistry: The Ritual Persecution of Drugs, Addicts, and Pushers*; Szasz, *Our Right to Drugs: The Case for a Free Market.*

24. Roy Porter, *A Social History of Madness,* 6; Nancy C. Andreasen, "DSM and the Death of Phenomenology in America: An Example of Unintended Consequences."

1. Malingering

1. H. Gavin, *On Feigned and Factitious Diseases Chiefly of Soldiers and Seamen, on the Means Used to Simulate or Produce Them, and on the Best Modes of Detecting Impostors.*

2. Ibid., i, vii.

3. Ibid., 10.

4. Jan E. Goldstein, *Console and Classify: The French Psychiatric Profession in the Nineteenth Century,* 234.

5. The process of renaming autogenic behaviors to conceal the agency of the self began earlier, with the replacing of terms such as *self-murder* and *self-slaughter* with the term *suicide.*

6. Thomas Szasz, *Coercion as Cure: A Critical History of Psychiatry.*

7. Robert Brudenell Carter, *On the Pathology and Treatment of Hysteria,* 1–2.

8. John Selden quoted in K. Thomas, *Religion and the Decline of Magic,* 435.

9. The only language free of such prejudgment is mathematics: its terms are defined before or as they are used.

10. Carter, *Pathology and Treatment of Hysteria,* 94, 93.

11. Feuchtersleben, *Principles of Medical Psychology,* 74–75.

12. Sigmund Freud, "Report on My Studies in Paris and Berlin" (1886), in *SE,* 1:5.

13. Ibid., 10, 11, 13 (emphasis added).

14. Henri F. Ellenberger, *The Discovery of the Unconscious: The History and Evolution of Dynamic Psychiatry,* 96–97 (emphasis added).

15. Freud, "Report on My Studies," in *SE,* 1:13 (emphasis added).

16. Ernst Kretschmer quoted in Kurt R. Eissler, *Freud as an Expert Witness: The Discussion of War Neuroses Between Freud and Wagner-Jauregg,* 340.

17. See Thomas Szasz, *The Ethics of Psychoanalysis: The Theory and Method of Autonomous Psychotherapy.*

18. Sigmund Freud, *Introductory Lectures on Psychoanalysis* (1915–1917), in *SE,* 16:457.

19. In English we "have" dreams, but in French we "make" them *(faire des rêves).*

20. Kurt R. Eissler, "Malingering," 252–53.

21. Phillip J. Resnick and J. Knoll, "Faking It: How to Detect Malingered Psychosis," 16; Victor Kuperman, "Narratives of Psychiatric Malingering in Works of Fiction," 67–72 (emphasis added).

22. K. Horrigan, "In Iraq as in World War II, Soldiers' Wounds Go Well Beyond the Physical," *Syracuse Post-Standard,* Nov. 25, 2007, E1.

23. T. Preid, "Teen Boys at Growing Risk for Eating Disorders," http://body.aol.com/news/health/article/_a/teen-boys-at-growing-risk-for-eating/20071126112909990001.

24. See Szasz, *Coercion as Cure,* 106–8.

25. Quoted in J. M. S. Pearce, "Silas Weir Mitchell and the 'Rest Cure,'" 381, available at http://jnnp.bmjjournals.com/cgi/content/full/75/3/381.

26. "Silas Weir Mitchell," http://www.whonamedit.com/doctor.cfm/959.html.

27. Josef Breuer, "Theoretical," in *SE*, 2:185; Breuer, "Theoretisches," in *Gesammelte Werke, Nachtragsband: Texte aus den Jahren, 1885–1938,* by Sigmund Freud, 287.

28. Breuer, "Theoretical," in *SE*, 2:227–28; Breuer, "Theoretisches," in *Gesammelte Werke, Nachtragsband,* by Freud, 287.

29. Karin Stephen, *The Wish to Fall Ill: A Study of Psychoanalysis and Medicine,* 1 (emphasis in the original).

30. Ibid., 4 (emphasis added).

31. Ibid.

32. Ibid., 5 (emphasis added).

33. Ibid., 7.

34. Ibid., 27 (emphasis added).

35. http://www.enotes.com/famous-quotes/the-diagnosis-of-drunkenness-was-that-it-was-a.

36. Thomas Szasz, *Anti-Freud: Karl Kraus's Criticism of Psychoanalysis and Psychiatry*; H. L. Mencken, "Studies of Vulgar Psychology: The Art Eternal," *New York Evening Mail,* 1918; Mencken, *Prejudices: Fourth Series*; http://www.mencken.org/text/txt001/elliott.leo.1998.mencken-01.htm.

37. Karl Jaspers, *General Psychopathology,* 329.

38. Ibid., 423.

39. Ibid., 424. In this connection, see Chapter 6.

40. Anna Freud, *Normality and Pathology in Childhood: Assessments of Development,* 120.

41. Sigmund Freud, *The Question of Lay Analysis* (1927), in *SE*, 20:229; Freud, *New Introductory Lectures on Psychoanalysis* (1932–1936), in *SE*, 22:153, 152.

42. Freud, *New Introductory Lectures,* in *SE*, 22:252, 230; Freud, "An Outline of Psychoanalysis" (1940), in *SE*, 23:77.

2. Doctoring

1. Ernest-Charles Lasègue quoted in Georges Guillain, *J.-M. Charcot, 1823–1893: His Life—His Work,* 324. See also "Lasègue's Sign," http://www.whonamedit.com/synd.cfm/2468.html. Georges Gilles de la Tourette quoted in Georges Didi-Huberman, *The Invention of Hysteria: Charcot and the Photographic Iconography of the Salpêtrière,* 293.

2. Goldstein, *Console and Classify,* 84.

3. Émile Zola quoted in ibid., 381.

4. Guillain, *J.-M. Charcot,* 87–88.

5. "Seeing Is Believing," in *Iconographie photographique de la Salpêtrière, Service de M. Charcot* (Paris: Bureau du Progrès Médical, V. Adrien Delahay et Cie, 1877–1880), Photography Collection, Miriam and Ira D. Wallach Division of Art, Prints, and Photographs, the New York Public Library, http://seeing.nypl.org/198t.html.

6. James Strachey, "Editor's Note," in "Charcot" (1893), in *SE*, 3:9–10.

7. Sigmund Freud, "Hysteria" (1888), in *SE*, 1:41 (emphasis added).

8. Ibid., 50.

9. Ibid., 52, 54.

10. Freud, "Charcot," in *SE*, 3:12–13.

11. Sigmund Freud, "Preface and Footnotes to the Translation of Charcot's Tuesday Lectures" (1892), in *SE*, 1:135–36.

12. Sigmund Freud, "Some Points for a Comparative Study of Organic and Hysterical Motor Paralyses" (1893), in *SE*, 1:162, 169 (emphases in the original); Freud, "Charcot," in *SE*, 3:22.

13. Guillain, *J.-M. Charcot*, 174; Freud, "Charcot," in *SE*, 3:22.

14. Quoted in Guillain, *J.-M. Charcot*, 56.

15. Ibid., 136–37.

16. Ibid., 138–39.

17. Ibid., 139.

18. Ibid., 142.

19. Ibid.

20. Ibid., 174.

21. Ibid., 175–76.

22. Ibid., 176.

23. Ibid., 147–48.

24. Quoted in ibid., 149 (emphasis added).

25. Axel Munthe, *The Story of San Michele*, 284–85.

26. Ibid., 303.

27. Ibid., 312–13.

28. Ibid., 314.

29. The terms *hypnosis* and *hypnotism* were coined by James Braid (1795–1860), a Scottish surgeon, in 1843, when he found that some subjects went into a "trance" by fixating their eyes on a bright object, like a silver watch. He believed that the phenomenon was similar to natural sleep, hence the name, and that some sort of neurophysiological process was involved in its production. Subsequently, French neurologist Hippolyte Bernheim (1837–1919), a professor at the University of Nancy, became the leader of hypnosis as a special form of sleeping where the subject's attention is focused on the suggestions made by the hypnotist. Although he emphasized the psychological nature of the process, he was instrumental in establishing hypnotism as a medical procedure, unsafe in the hands of the nonphysician.

30. Ibid., 322.

31. Silas Weir Mitchell, "Address Before the Fiftieth Annual Meeting of the American Medico-Psychological Association, Held in Philadelphia, May 16th, 1894," 414, 427 (emphasis added).

3. Inculpating

1. William James, "A Plea for Psychology as a Natural Science," 146.

2. Sigmund Freud, *The Psychopathology of Everyday Life* (1901), in *SE*, 6:254.

3. Freud, *An Outline of Psychoanalysis,* in *SE*, 23:158; Freud, *Gesammelte Werke*, 17:80 (emphasis added).

4. Freud, *An Outline of Psychoanalysis,* in *SE*, 23:163, 196; Freud, *Gesammelte Werke,* 17:86, 119.

5. Sigmund Freud, "Some Elementary Lessons in Psychoanalysis" (1938), in *SE*, 23:282.

6. M. Sharaf, *Fury on Earth: A Biography of Wilhelm Reich.*

7. Sigmund Freud, "On the History of the Psycho-analytic Movement" (1914), in *SE*, 14:21–22, 38. Christian Friedrich Hebbel (1813–1863) was a German poet and dramatist.

8. Sigmund Freud, "A Difficulty in the Path of Psychoanalysis" (1917), in *SE*, 17:135–44.

9. Jean-Paul Sartre, *Being and Nothingness: An Essay on Phenomenological Ontology,* 51.

10. Freud, "Difficulty in the Path," in *SE*, 17:141–42.

11. See Szasz, *Anti-Freud.*

12. Sigmund Freud, "Case 5: Fräulein Elisabeth von R.," in *Studies on Hysteria* (1893–1895), by Josef Breuer and Sigmund Freud, in *SE*, 2:160–61.

13. Sigmund Freud, "The Claims of Psychoanalysis to Scientific Interest" (1913), in *SE*, 13:176.

14. Thomas Szasz, *The Meaning of Mind: Language, Morality, and Neuroscience,* 17.

15. Bruno Bettelheim, *Freud and Man's Soul,* 15–16.

16. Ibid., 40–41.

17. See Jacques Barzun, *Science: The Glorious Entertainment.*

18. Bettelheim, *Freud and Man's Soul,* 43.

19. Freud, *New Introductory Lectures,* in *SE,* 22:158–60 (emphasis added).

20. Freud, *Introductory Lectures on Psychoanalysis,* in *SE,* 16:27, 28.

21. Ibid. 49, 106.

22. Jean-Paul Sartre, *Sketch for a Theory of the Emotions,* 54 (emphasis in the original); Sartre, *Being and Nothingness,* 51.

23. Adam Kirsch, "The Unreliable Superego," July 31, 2003, http://www.slate.com/id/2086413/.

24. See Thomas Szasz, "Freud as a Leader."

25. Stanley Edgar Hyman, *The Tangled Bank: Darwin, Marx, Frazer, and Freud as Imaginative Writers,* 313.

26. Sigmund Freud, "Psychoanalysis and the Establishment of the Facts in Legal Proceedings" (1906), in *SE,* 9:108; Hyman, *Tangled Bank,* 302.

27. Hyman, *Tangled Bank,* 313; Sigmund Freud, "The Moses of Michelangelo" (1914), in *SE,* 13:222.

28. Stefan Zweig, "Portrait of Freud" (1932), 93, an excerpt from Zweig's *Mental Healers: Franz Anton Mesmer, Mary Baker Eddy, Sigmund Freud*; Thomas Mann quoted in R. W. Clark, *Freud: The Man and the Cause*, 418.

29. See Thomas Szasz, *The Myth of Psychotherapy: Mental Healing as Religion, Rhetoric, and Repression*; and Szasz, *Insanity*.

30. Carlo Ginzburg, "Morelli, Freud, and Sherlock Holmes: Clues and Scientific Method," 81.

31. Ibid., 88–89.

32. Ibid., 92 (emphasis in the original).

33. Freud, "The Moses of Michelangelo," in *SE*, 13:211.

34. Marcello Truzzi, "Sherlock Holmes: Applied Social Scientist," 74.

4. Sheltering

1. Karl Wernicke quoted in E. J. Engstrom, *Clinical Psychiatry in Imperial Germany: A History of Psychiatric Practice*, 251.

2. See Szasz, *Insanity*; and Szasz, *Cruel Compassion: The Psychiatric Control of Society's Unwanted*.

3. Brooke Kroeger, *Nellie Bly: Daredevil, Reporter, Feminist*, 85–86.

4. Nellie Bly, *Ten Days in a Mad-House*. All quotes are from http://digital.library.upenn.edu/women/bly/madhouse/madhouse.html (emphases added).

5. See Thomas Szasz, *Ideology and Insanity: Essays on the Psychiatric Dehumanization of Man*.

6. Eissler, *Freud as an Expert Witness*, xii.

7. Ibid., xvi.

8. Ibid., xvi, 15.

9. Ibid., 21.

10. Sigmund Freud, "Appendix: Memorandum on the Electrical Treatment of War Neuroses"; Eissler, *Freud as an Expert Witness*, 23–28. My references to the memorandum are from Eissler's text.

11. Ibid., 28 (emphasis added).

12. Ibid., 25–26 (emphasis added).

13. Ibid., 26 (emphasis added).

14. Ibid., 26–27 (emphasis added), 28 (emphasis added).

15. Sigmund Freud, introduction to *Psychoanalysis and the War Neuroses* (1919), 209; Freud, "Memorandum on the Electrical Treatment of War Neurotics" (1920), in *SE*, 17:213.

16. David L. Rosenhan, "On Being Sane in Insane Places," available at http://web.cocc.edu/lminorevans/on_being_sane_in_insane_places.htm; and http://www.sciencemag.org/cgi/content/abstract/179/4070/250. Subsequent quotes are from this source.

17. See Thomas Szasz, "The Lying Truths of Psychiatry," 121–42.

18. See Thomas Szasz, "The Myth of Mental Illness"; and Szasz, *Myth of Mental Illness.*

19. David L. Rosenhan and Martin E. P. Seligman, *Abnormal Psychology,* 604–5, 616.

20. Szasz, "Lying Truths of Psychiatry," 121–42 (emphasis added).

21. Roy Porter, introduction to *The Confinement of the Insane: International Perspectives, 1800–1965,* edited by Roy Porter and D. Wright, 2.

22. Donald Naftulin et al., "The Doctor Fox Lecture: A Paradigm of Educational Seduction." Subsequent quotes are from this source.

23. In this connection, see "The Sokal Affair" and "Science Wars," in *Fashionable Nonsense: Postmodern Intellectuals' Abuse of Science,* by Alan Sokal and Jean Bricmont; and "Fashionable Nonsense," http://en.wikipedia.org/wiki/Fashionable_Nonsense.

24. "Transcript of the German TV Reportage on the Postel Experiment, 7.06.'07," http://www.gert-postel.de/english.htm; http://www.iaapa.de/halli_kalli.html; http://www.gert-postel.de/io_anniversary_speech.htm.

5. Cheating

1. Associated Press, "German Pole-Vaulter Yvonne Buschbaum Retires, Plans Hormone Treatment," Nov. 21, 2007, http://www.iht.com/articles/ap/2007/11/21/sports/EU-SPT-ATH-Buschbaum-Retires.php; M. D. Smith, "Pole Vaulter Yvonne Buschbaum Retires, Plans to Change Genders," Nov. 22, 2007, http://sports.aol.com/fanhouse/2007/11/22/pole-vaulter-yvonne-buschbaum-retires-plans-to-change-genders/?ncid=NWS00010000000001.

2. For example, see A. L. Cowan, "Suit over a Woman's Suicide at an Elite Private Hospital," *New York Times,* Nov. 23, 2007, http://www.nytimes.com/2007/11/23/nyregion/23psych.html.

3. John Godley, *Van Meegeren: A Case History;* F. Wynne, *I Was Vermeer: The Legend of the Forger Who Swindled the Nazis.* See also http://en.wikipedia.org/wiki/Han_van_Meegeren.

4. Thomas Szasz, "An Autobiographical Sketch," in *Szasz under Fire: The Psychiatric Abolitionist Faces His Critics,* edited by J. A. Schaler, 1–28.

5. R. O. Pasnau, "The Remedicalization of Psychiatry." See also M. Sabshin, "On Remedicalization and Holism in Psychiatry."

6. Mary G. Baker and Matthew Menken, "Time to Abandon the Term Mental Illness," 937 (emphasis added).

7. See Guy A. Boysen, "An Evaluation of the DSM Concept of Mental Disorder."

8. Ibid.

9. White House Press Office, *White House Fact Sheet on Myths and Facts about Mental Illness,* June 5, 1999; President Clinton quoted in "Myths and Facts about Mental Illness," *New York Times,* June 7, 1999, Internet edition (see also http://www.info@ariannaonline.com); Tipper Gore quoted in Office of the Press Secretary of the President of the United States, "Remarks by the President, the First Lady, the Vice President, and Mrs. Gore at White House Conference on Mental Health," Blackburn Auditorium, June 7, 1999, Howard Univ.,

Washington, D.C.; "Satcher Discusses MH Issues Hurting Black Community," 6; Nancy C. Andreasen, "What Is Psychiatry?"

10. R. Wyatt, "An Essay by Dr. Richard Wyatt," ESI Special Topics, Dec. 2001, http://www.esitopics.com/schizophrenia/interviews/Dr-Richard-Wyatt.html. Subsequent quotes are from this source.

11. S. G. Potkin et al., "Are Paranoid Schizophrenics Biologically Different from Other Schizophrenics?"; P. A. Berger et al., "Platelet Monoamine Oxidase in Chronic Schizophrenic Patients."

12. K. Pajari, "Monoamine Oxidase in Schizophrenia" (letters), *New England Journal of Medicine* 298 (May 18, 1978): 1150; Potkin et al., letter, *New England Journal of Medicine* 298 (May 18, 1978): 1151–52.

13. Editors, "Schizophrenia and Publication," *New England Journal of Medicine* 298 (May 18, 1978): 1152.

14. J. Rosack, "Patient Charged with Murder of Schizophrenia Expert," 1, 7, http://pn.psychiatryonline.org/cgi/content/full/41/19/1. Subsequent quotes are from this source.

6. Lying

1. J. Morgan, "Tipper Gore Honors Mental Health Achievements," http://www.usatoday.com/news/health/spotlighthealth/2003-05-20-gore.htm.

2. "Betty Ford," http://en.wikipedia.org/wiki/Betty_Ford.

3. "Clifford Whittingham Beers," http://en.wikipedia.org/wiki/Clifford_Whittingham_Beers.

4. http://www.cliffordbeers.org/clifford.w.beers.htm.

5. "Kay Redfield Jamison," http://en.wikipedia.org/wiki/Kay_Redfield_Jamison.

6. "Dr. Kay Jamison's Near-Death Experience: Kevin Williams' NDE and Mental Illness Research," http://www.near-death.com/experiences/triggers22.html. For further analysis of Jamison's views, see Thomas Szasz, *"My Madness Saved Me": The Madness and Marriage of Virginia Woolf,* 98–110.

7. Lauren Slater, *Lying: A Metaphorical Memoir,* 219–20.

8. Ibid., 6.

9. Ibid., 5–6.

10. Ibid., 60.

11. Ibid., 170, 169.

12. Ibid., 159–65 (emphasis in the original); http://www.whatquote.com/quotes/Mary-Mccarthy/28155-Every-word-she-write.htm.

13. Slater, *Lying,* 161, 163.

14. Ibid., 166–67.

15. http://www.amazon.com/Welcome-My-Country-Lauren-Slater/dp/0385487398/ref=sr_1_1/103-8560227-0826219?ie=UTF8&s=books&qid=1188964229&sr=8-1.

16. Lauren Slater, *Opening Skinner's Box: Great Psychological Experiments of the Twentieth Century*, 1.

17. Ibid., 3 (emphasis added).

18. Ibid.

19. Ibid., 65, 73 (emphasis in the original).

20. Ibid., 73.

21. Ibid., 67.

22. Ibid., 80–81 (emphasis added).

23. Ibid., 83.

24. See Szasz, *Cruel Compassion*.

25. Slater, *Opening Skinner's Box*, 83.

26. Ibid., 88–89 (emphasis added).

27. Ibid., 93.

28. Mark Moran, "Writer Ignites Firestorm with Misdiagnosis Claims," 10, http://pn.psychiatryonline.org/cgi/content/full/41/7/10. Subsequent references are to this source.

29. http://en.wikipedia.org/wiki/Pseudologia_fantastica.

30. "Pseudologia Fantastica: A Brief 21st Century History of Résumé Fraud," http://mayorsam.blogspot.com/2006/05/pseudologia-fantastica-brief-21st.html.

31. "Impostor Syndrome," http://en.wikipedia.org/wiki/Impostor_Syndrome.

32. http://www.impostorsyndrome.com/.

33. Oscar Wilde, *The Importance of Being Earnest: A Trivial Comedy for Serious People*, act 1, pt. 1, http://www.hoboes.com/html/FireBlade/Wilde/earnest/.

Epilogue: The Burden of Responsibility

1. Jaspers, *General Psychopathology*, 425 (emphasis in the original).

2. Friedrich Nietzsche, *Twilight of the Idols; or, How to Philosophize with a Hammer*, 505 (emphasis in the original).

3. Lord Acton, "Acton-Creighton Correspondence: Letter to Mandell Creighton, April 5, 1887," in *Essays in the Study and Writing of History*, by J. E. E. D. Acton, 2:383.

4. Lord Acton, "Acton and Döllinger: Letter to Johann Joseph Ignaz Döllinger, June 16, 1882," in ibid., 3:666.

5. Ibid., 667–70.

6. Ibid., 672.

7. Damien McElrath and James Holland, preface to *Lord Acton: The Decisive Decade, 1864–1874; Essays and Documents*, by Damien McElrath et al., vii–ix, 23, 41 (emphasis added).

8. Szasz, introduction to *Ideology and Insanity*, 11.

9. Thomas Jefferson, "Notes on the State of Virginia" (1782). Compilation copyrighted 1996 by Eyler Robert Coates Sr. Permission hereby granted to quote single excerpts separately; http://etext.virginia.edu/jefferson/quotations/jeff3.htm.

Bibliography

Abbott, C. *Forging Fame: The Strange Career of Scharmel Iris.* DeKalb: Northern Illinois Univ. Press, 2007.

Ackerknecht, Erwin H. *Rudolf Virchow: Doctor, Statesman, Anthropologist.* Madison: Univ. of Wisconsin Press, 1953.

Acton, J. E. E. D. *Essays in the Study and Writing of History.* Edited by J. Rufus Fears. 3 vols. Indianapolis: Liberty Classics, 1988.

Andreasen, Nancy C. "DSM and the Death of Phenomenology in America: An Example of Unintended Consequences." *Schizophrenia Bulletin* 33 (2007): 108–12.

———. "What Is Psychiatry?" *American Journal of Psychiatry* 154 (May 1997): 591–93.

Andreski, S. *Social Sciences as Sorcery.* Harmondsworth: Penguin, 1974.

———. *Syphilis, Puritanism, and Witch Hunts: Historical Explanation in the Light of Medicine and Psychoanalysis with a Forecast about AIDS.* New York: St. Martin's Press, 1989.

Baker, Mary G., and Matthew Menken. "Time to Abandon the Term Mental Illness." *British Medical Journal* 322 (2001).

Baritz, Loren. *The Servants of Power: A History of the Use of Social Sciences in American Industry.* Middletown, Conn.: Wesleyan Univ. Press, 1960.

Barnes, John A. *A Pack of Lies: Toward a Sociology of Lying.* Cambridge: Cambridge Univ. Press, 1994.

Barzun, Jacques. *Science: The Glorious Entertainment.* New York: Harper and Row, 1964.

Beers, Clifford Whittingham. *A Mind That Found Itself: An Autobiography.* 7th ed. 1908. Reprint, Garden City, N.Y.: Doubleday, 1956.

Berger, P. A., et al., "Platelet Monoamine Oxidase in Chronic Schizophrenic Patients." *American Journal of Psychiatry* 135 (Jan. 1978): 95–99.

Bettelheim, Bruno. *Freud and Man's Soul.* New York: Alfred A. Knopf, 1983.

Bierce, Ambrose. *The Unabridged Devil's Dictionary*. Edited by D. E. Schultz and S. T. Joshi. Athens: Univ. of Georgia Press, 2000.

Bleuler, E. *A Textbook of Psychiatry*. Translated by A. A. Brill. 1924. Reprint, New York: Macmillan, 1944.

Bly, Nellie. *Ten Days in a Mad-House*. Published with "Miscellaneous Sketches: Trying to Be a Servant" and "Nellie Bly as a White Slave." 1887. Reprint, New York: Ian L. Munro, n.d.

Bok, Sissela. *Lying: Moral Choice in Public and Private Life*. New York: Vintage, 1979.

Boysen, Guy A. "An Evaluation of the DSM Concept of Mental Disorder." *Journal of Mind and Behavior* 28 (2007): 157–74.

Breuer, Josef, and Sigmund Freud. *Studies on Hysteria*. In vol. 2 of *The Standard Edition of the Complete Psychological Works of Sigmund Freud*, translated by James Strachey. 24 vols. 1893–1895. Reprint, London: Hogarth Press, 1953–1974.

Brissett, D., and C. Edgley, eds. *Life as Theater: A Dramaturgical Sourcebook*. 2d ed. New York: Aldine de Gruyter, 1990.

Burke, P., and Roy Porter, eds. *The Social History of Language*. Cambridge: Cambridge Univ. Press, 1987.

Canguilhem, G. *On the Normal and the Pathological*. Boston: D. Reidel, 1978.

Carter, Robert Brudenell. *On the Pathology and Treatment of Hysteria*. London: John Churchill, 1853.

Cioffi, F. *Freud and the Question of Pseudoscience*. Chicago: Open Court, 1999.

Clark, R. D. *Freud: The Man and the Cause*. London: Jonathan Cape and Weidenfeld and Nicolson, 1980.

Danto, Elizabeth Ann. *Freud's Free Clinics: Psychoanalysis and Social Justice, 1918–1938*. New York: Columbia Univ. Press, 2005.

DeGrandpre, Richard. *The Cult of Pharmacology: How America Became the World's Most Troubled Drug Culture*. Durham: Duke Univ. Press, 2006.

Didi-Huberman, Georges. *The Invention of Hysteria: Charcot and the Photographic Iconography of the Salpêtrière*. Translated by Alisa Hartz. 1982. Reprint, Cambridge: MIT Press, 2004.

Drinka, G. F. *The Birth of Neurosis: Myth, Malady, and the Victorians*. New York: Simon and Schuster, 1984.

Eco, U., and T. Sebeok, eds. *The Sign of Three: Dupin, Holmes, Peirce*. Bloomington: Indiana Univ. Press, 1983.

Eissler, Kurt R. *Freud as an Expert Witness: The Discussion of War Neuroses Between Freud and Wagner-Jauregg*. Translated by Christine Trollope. Madison, Conn.: International Universities Press, 1986.

———. "Malingering." In *Psychoanalysis and Culture,* edited by G. B. Wilbur and W. Muensterberger. New York: International Universities Press, 1951.

———, ed. *Searchlights on Delinquency: New Psychoanalytic Studies.* New York: International Universities Press, 1949.

Ellenberger, Henri F. *The Discovery of the Unconscious: The History and Evolution of Dynamic Psychiatry.* New York: Basic Books, 1970.

Engstrom, E. J. *Clinical Psychiatry in Imperial Germany: A History of Psychiatric Practice.* Ithaca: Cornell Univ. Press, 2003.

Erichsen, J. E. *On Railway and Other Injuries of the Nervous System.* London: Walton and Maberly, 1866.

Fearnside, W. W., and W. B. Holther. *Fallacy: The Counterfeit Argument.* Englewood Cliffs, N.J.: Prentice-Hall, 1959.

Feinstein, Alvan R. *Clinical Judgment.* Baltimore: Williams and Wilkins, 1967.

Feuchtersleben, Ernst von. *The Dietetics of the Soul.* Unidentified translator. 1838. Reprint, New York: C. S. Francis, 1858. Originally published as *Zur Diätetik der Seele.*

———. *Hygiene of the Mind.* Translated by F. C. Sumner. 1838. Reprint, New York: Macmillan, 1933. Originally published as *Zur Diätetik der Seele.*

———. *The Principles of Medical Psychology, Being the Outline of a Course of Lectures.* Translated by H. Evans Lloyd. 1835. Reprint, London: Printed for the Sydenham Society, 1847.

Feynman, Richard P., and R. Leighton. *What Do You Care What Other People Think? Further Adventures of a Curious Character.* New York: W. W. Norton, 2001.

Frankfurt, H. G. *On Bullshit.* Princeton: Princeton Univ. Press, 2005.

Freud, Anna. *Normality and Pathology in Childhood: Assessments of Development.* New York: International Universities Press, 1965.

Freud, Sigmund. "Appendix: Memorandum on the Electrical Treatment of War Neuroses." 1920. In *SE,* 17:211–15.

———. "An Autobiographical Study." 1924. In *SE* 20.

———. "The Claims of Psychoanalysis to Scientific Interest." 1913. In *SE* 13.

———. *The Complete Letters of Sigmund Freud to Wilhelm Fliess, 1887–1904.* Edited by Jeffrey M. Masson. Cambridge: Harvard Univ. Press, 1986.

———. "Five Lectures on Psychoanalysis." 1909. In *SE* 11.

———. "Future Prospects of Psychoanalytic Therapy." 1910. In *SE* 11.

———. *Gesammelte Werke.* 18 vols. Frankfurt am Main: S. Fischer, 1960–1968.

———. *Gesammelte Werke, Nachtragsband: Texte aus den Jahren, 1885–1938.* Frankfurt am Main: S. Fischer, 1987.

———. Introduction to *Psychoanalysis and the War Neuroses*. 1919. In *SE*, 17:205–10.

———. *Introductory Lectures on Psychoanalysis*. 1915–1917. In *SE* 16.

———. *New Introductory Lectures on Psychoanalysis*. 1932–1936. In *SE* 22.

———. "On Beginning the Treatment." 1913. In *SE* 12.

———. "On the History of the Psycho-analytic Movement." 1914. In *SE* 14.

———. "An Outline of Psychoanalysis." 1940. In *SE* 23.

———. *The Psychopathology of Everyday Life*. 1901. In *SE* 6 (1901).

———. *The Standard Edition of the Complete Psychological Works of Sigmund Freud*. 24 vols. London: Hogarth Press, 1953–1974.

Friedman, Lawrence J. *Identity's Architect: A Biography of Erik H. Erikson*. New York: Scribner, 1999.

Gavin, H. *On Feigned and Factitious Diseases Chiefly of Soldiers and Seamen, on the Means Used to Simulate or Produce Them, and on the Best Modes of Detecting Impostors*. London: John Churchill, 1843.

Gay, P. *Freud: A Life for Our Time*. New York: W. W. Norton, 1988.

Gilman, S. L., H. King, R. Porter, G. S. Rousseau, and E. Showalter. *Hysteria Beyond Freud*. Berkeley and Los Angeles: Univ. of California Press, 1993.

Ginzburg, Carlo. "Morelli, Freud, and Sherlock Holmes: Clues and Scientific Method." In *The Sign of Three: Dupin, Holmes, Peirce*, edited by U. Eco and T. Sebeok, 81–118. Bloomington: Indiana Univ. Press, 1983.

Godley, John. *Master Art Forger: The Story of Han van Meegeren*. New York: Wilfred Funk, 1951.

———. *Van Meegeren: A Case History*. London: Thomas Nelson and Sons, 1967.

Goldberg, M. Hirsh. *The Book of Lies: History's Greatest Fakes, Frauds, Schemes, and Scams*. New York: Quill / William Morrow, 1990.

Goldstein, Jan E. *Console and Classify: The French Psychiatric Profession in the Nineteenth Century*. Cambridge: Cambridge Univ. Press, 1987.

Gorky, M. *"The Lower Depths," and Other Plays*. Translated by Alexander Bakshy. New Haven: Yale Univ. Press, 1945.

Guillain, Georges. *J.-M. Charcot, 1823–1893: His Life—His Work*. Translated by Pearce Bailey. New York: Paul B. Hoeber, 1959.

Halligan, Peter W., Christopher Bass, and David A. Oakley, eds. *Malingering and Illness Deception*. Oxford: Oxford Univ. Press, 2003.

Hunter, R., and I. Macalpine, eds. *Three Hundred Years of Psychiatry, 1535–1860: A History Presented in Selected English Texts*. London: Oxford Univ. Press, 1963.

Hyman, Stanley Edgar. *The Tangled Bank: Darwin, Marx, Frazer, and Freud as Imaginative Writers.* New York: Atheneum, 1962.

Jackson, J. H. *Selected Writings of John Hughlings Jackson.* Edited by James Taylor. 2 vols. London: Staples Press, 1958.

James, William. "A Plea for Psychology as a Natural Science." *Philosophical Reviews* 1 (1892): 146–53.

———. *The Varieties of Religious Experience: A Study in Human Nature.* 1902. Reprint, New York: Mentor Books, 1958.

Janet, Pierre. *The Major Symptoms of Hysteria: Fifteen Lectures Given in the Medical School of Harvard University.* 2d ed. 1906. Reprint, New York: Macmillan, 1920.

———. *The Mental State of Hystericals: A Study of Mental Stigmata and Mental Accidents.* With a preface by Professor J.-M. Charcot. Translated by Caroline Rollin Corson. New York: G. P. Putnam's Sons, 1901. Reprinted in *Significant Contributions to the History of Psychology, 1750–1920,* edited with an introduction by Daniel N. Robinson. Washington, D.C.: University Publications of America, 1977.

———. *Psychological Healing: A Historical and Clinical Study.* Translated by Eden Paul and Cedar Paul. 2 vols. New York: Macmillan, 1925.

Jaspers, Karl. *General Psychopathology.* 7th ed. Translated by J. Hoenig and M. W. Hamilton. 1913. Reprint, Chicago: Univ. of Chicago Press, 1963.

Jones, E. *The Life and Works of Sigmund Freud.* 3 vols. New York: Basic Books, 1953–1957.

Jung, C. G. *The Collected Works of C. G. Jung.* Translated by R. F. C. Hull. Edited by H. Read et al. 21 vols. Princeton: Princeton Univ. Press, 1953–2000.

———. *Memories, Dreams, Reflections.* Edited by Aniela Jaffé. Translated by Richard and Clara Winston. New York: Pantheon Books, 1961.

Krafft-Ebing, Richard von. *Psychopathia Sexualis, with Special Reference to the Antipathic Sexual Instinct: A Medico-Forensic Study.* 1886. Authorized English adaptation of the twelfth German edition by F. J. Rebman (1906). Rev. ed. Brooklyn: Physicians and Surgeons Book Company, 1931.

Kretschmer, Ernst. *Hysteria, Reflex, and Instinct.* 1923. Reprint, New York: Philosophical Library, 1960.

———. *Hysterie, Reflex, und Instinkt.* 6th ed. 1923. Reprint, Stuttgart: Georg Thieme Verlag, 1958.

Kroeger, Brooke. *Nellie Bly: Daredevil, Reporter, Feminist.* New York: Random House / Times Books, 1994.

Kuperman, Victor. "Narratives of Psychiatric Malingering in Works of Fiction." *Journal of Medical Ethics/Medical Humanities* 32 (2006): 67–72.

Lerner, Paul. *Hysterical Men: War, Psychiatry, and the Politics of Trauma in Germany, 1890–1930*. Ithaca: Cornell Univ. Press, 2003.

Letwin, Shirley Robin. *The Pursuit of Certainty: David Hume, Jeremy Bentham, John Stuart Mill, Beatrice Webb*. Indianapolis: Liberty Fund, 1998.

Libbrecht, Katrien. *Hysterical Psychosis: A Historical Survey*. New Brunswick, N.J.: Transaction Publishers, 1995.

MacFarquhar, L. "Bag Man: Cracking Down on Fashion Fakes." *New Yorker*, Mar. 19, 2007, 126–35.

Magnusson, M. *Fakers, Forgers, and Phoneys: Famous Scams and Scamps*. London: Mainstream, 2007.

Maines, Rachel P. *The Technology of Orgasm: "Hysteria," the Vibrator, and Women's Sexual Satisfaction*. Baltimore: Johns Hopkins Univ. Press, 1999.

Malcolm, J. *In the Freud Archives*. 1984. Reprint, New York: Granta, 2004.

McElrath, Damien, James Holland, W. White, and S. Katzman. *Lord Acton: The Decisive Decade, 1864–1874; Essays and Documents*. Louvain, Belgium: Publications Universitaires de Louvain, 1970.

McNeill, John T. *A History of the Cure of Souls*. New York: Harper Torchbooks, 1951.

Mencken, H. L. *Prejudices: Fourth Series*. New York: Alfred A. Knopf, 1924.

Meynert, T. *Psychiatry: Clinical Treatise on Diseases of the Forebrain*. Translated by B. Sachs. 1884. Reprint, New York: G. P. Putnam's Sons, 1985.

Micale, Mark S. "Hysteria and Its Historiography: The Future Perspective." *History of Psychiatry* 1 (1990): 33–124.

Micale, Mark S., and Paul Lerner, eds. *Traumatic Pasts: History, Psychiatry, and Trauma in the Modern Age, 1870–1930*. Cambridge: Cambridge Univ. Press, 2001.

Mitchell, Silas Weir. "Address Before the Fiftieth Annual Meeting of the American Medico-Psychological Association, Held in Philadelphia, May 16th, 1894." *Journal of Nervous and Mental Disease* 21 (July 1894): 413–37.

———. *Fat and Blood; or, Hints for the Overworked*. Philadelphia: J. B. Lippincott, 1878. Edited and introduced by Michael S. Kimmel. Reprint, Walnut Creek, Calif.: Altamira Press, 2004.

Moran, M. "Writer Ignites Firestorm with Misdiagnosis Claims." *Psychiatric News* 41 (Apr. 7, 2006).

Munthe, Axel. *The Story of San Michele*. New York: Dutton, 1929.

Naftulin, Donald, et al. "The Doctor Fox Lecture: A Paradigm of Educational Seduction." *Journal of Medical Education* 48 (July 1973): 630–35.

New Cassell's German Dictionary: German-English, English-German. Edited by Harold T. Betteridge. New York: Funk and Wagnalls, 1958.

Nietzsche, Friedrich. *Twilight of the Idols; or, How to Philosophize with a Hammer*. In *The Portable Nietzsche,* edited and translated by Walter Kaufman. 1895. Reprint, New York: Viking, 1954.

Parrish, R. H. *Defining Drugs: How Government Became the Arbiter of Pharmaceutical Fact*. New Brunswick, N.J.: Transaction Publishers, 2003.

Pasnau, R. O. "The Remedicalization of Psychiatry." *Hospital and Community Psychiatry* 38 (Feb. 1987): 145–51.

Pearce, J. M. S. "Silas Weir Mitchell and the 'Rest Cure.'" *Journal of Neurology, Neurosurgery, and Psychiatry* 75 (2004).

Pickering, Neil. *The Metaphor of Mental Illness*. Oxford: Oxford Univ. Press, 2006.

Porter, Roy. *A Social History of Madness*. London: Weidenfeld and Nicolson, 1987.

Porter, Roy, and D. Wright, eds. *The Confinement of the Insane: International Perspectives, 1800–1965*. Cambridge: Cambridge Univ. Press, 2003.

Postel, G. *Doktorspiele: Geständnisse eines Hochstaplers* [Playing Doctor: Confessions of a Confidence Man]. Berlin: Eichborn, 2001.

Potkin, S. G., et al. "Are Paranoid Schizophrenics Biologically Different from Other Schizophrenics?" *New England Journal of Medicine* 298 (Jan. 12, 1978): 61–66.

Reese, David M. "Fundamentals: Rudolf Virchow and Modern Medicine." *Western Journal of Medicine* 169 (1998): 105–8.

Resnick, Phillip J., and J. Knoll. "Faking It: How to Detect Malingered Psychosis." *Current Psychiatry* 4 (Nov. 2005): 13–25.

Robitscher, Jonas. *The Powers of Psychiatry*. Boston: Houghton Mifflin, 1980.

Rosack, J. "Patient Charged with Murder of Schizophrenia Expert." *Psychiatric News* 41 (Oct. 6, 2006).

Rosenhan, David L. "On Being Sane in Insane Places." *Science* 179 (Jan. 19, 1973): 250–58.

Rosenhan, David L., and Martin E. P. Seligman. *Abnormal Psychology*. New York: W. W. Norton, 1984.

Rubin, Emanuel, and John L. Farber. *Pathology*. Philadelphia: Lippincott, 1994.

Ruitenbeek, H. M., ed. *Freud as We Knew Him*. Detroit: Wayne State Univ. Press, 1973.

Russell, B. *A History of Western Philosophy, and Its Connections with Political and Social Circumstances from the Earliest Times to the Present Day.* New York: Simon and Schuster, 1945.

Sabshin, M. "On Remedicalization and Holism in Psychiatry." *Psychosomatics* 18 (1977): 7–9.

Sartre, Jean-Paul. *Being and Nothingness: An Essay on Phenomenological Ontology.* Translated by Hazel E. Barnes. 1953. Reprint, New York: Philosophical Library, 1956.

———. *Sketch for a Theory of the Emotions.* Translated by Philip Mairet. 1939. Reprint, London: Methuen, 1962.

"Satcher Discusses MH Issues Hurting Black Community." *Psychiatric News* 34 (Oct. 15, 1999).

Schaler, J. A., ed. *Szasz under Fire: The Psychiatric Abolitionist Faces His Critics.* Chicago: Open Court, 2004.

Schreber, D. *Memoirs of My Nervous Illness.* Translated by Ida Macalpine and Richard Hunter. 1903. Reprint, London: William Dawson and Sons, 1955.

Schwartz, J. *Cassandra's Daughter: A History of Psychoanalysis.* New York: Viking, 1999.

Sharaf, M. *Fury on Earth: A Biography of Wilhelm Reich.* New York: St. Martin's Press, 1979.

Slater, Lauren. *Lying: A Metaphorical Memoir.* New York: Penguin, 2001.

———. *Opening Skinner's Box: Great Psychological Experiments of the Twentieth Century.* New York: W. W. Norton, 2004.

———. *Welcome to My Country: A Therapist's Memoir of Madness.* Random House / Anchor, 1997.

Sokal, Alan, and Jean Bricmont. *Fashionable Nonsense: Postmodern Intellectuals' Abuse of Science.* 1997. Reprint, New York: Picador, 1999.

Stephen, Karin. *The Wish to Fall Ill: A Study of Psychoanalysis and Medicine.* 1933. Reprint, Cambridge: Cambridge Univ. Press, 1960.

Sullivan, H. S. *The Interpersonal Theory of Psychiatry.* Edited by H. S. Perry and M. I. Gawell. New York: W. W. Norton, 1953.

Szasz, T. S. *Anti-Freud: Karl Kraus's Criticism of Psychoanalysis and Psychiatry.* 1976. Reprint, Syracuse: Syracuse Univ. Press, 1990.

———. "Bootlegging Humanistic Values Through Psychiatry." *Antioch Review* 22 (Fall 1962): 341–49.

———. *Ceremonial Chemistry: The Ritual Persecution of Drugs, Addicts, and Pushers.* Rev. ed. 1976. Reprint, Syracuse: Syracuse Univ. Press, 2003.

———. *Coercion as Cure: A Critical History of Psychiatry.* New Brunswick, N.J.: Transaction Publishers, 2007.

———. *Cruel Compassion: The Psychiatric Control of Society's Unwanted.* 1994. Reprint, Syracuse: Syracuse Univ. Press, 1998.

———. *The Ethics of Psychoanalysis: The Theory and Method of Autonomous Psychotherapy.* 1965. Reprint, Syracuse: Syracuse Univ. Press, 1988.

———. *Fatal Freedom: The Ethics and Politics of Suicide.* Westport, Conn.: Praeger, 1999.

———. "Freud as a Leader." *Antioch Review* 23 (Summer 1963): 133–44.

———. *Heresies.* Garden City, N.Y.: Doubleday-Anchor, 1976.

———. *Ideology and Insanity: Essays on the Psychiatric Dehumanization of Man.* 1970. Reprint, Syracuse: Syracuse Univ. Press, 1991.

———. *Insanity: The Idea and Its Consequences.* 1987. Reprint, Syracuse: Syracuse Univ. Press, 1997.

———. *Law, Liberty, and Psychiatry: An Inquiry into the Social Uses of Mental Health Practices.* 1963. Reprint, Syracuse: Syracuse Univ. Press, 1989.

———. *A Lexicon of Lunacy: Metaphoric Malady, Moral Responsibility, and Psychiatry.* New Brunswick, N.J.: Transaction Publishers, 1993.

———. *Liberation by Oppression: A Comparative Study of Slavery and Psychiatry.* New Brunswick, N.J.: Transaction Publishers, 2002.

———. "The Lying Truths of Psychiatry." In *Lying Truths: A Critical Scrutiny of Current Beliefs and Conventions,* edited by R. Duncan and M. Weston-Smith, 121–42. London: Pergamon Press, 1979.

———. "Malingering: 'Diagnosis' or Social Condemnation?" *AMA Archives of Neurology and Psychiatry* 76 (Oct. 1956): 432–43.

———. *The Manufacture of Madness: A Comparative Study of the Inquisition and the Mental Health Movement.* 1970. Reprint, Syracuse: Syracuse Univ. Press, 1997.

———. *The Meaning of Mind: Language, Morality, and Neuroscience.* 1996. Reprint, Syracuse: Syracuse Univ. Press, 2002.

———. *The Medicalization of Everyday Life: Selected Essays.* Syracuse: Syracuse Univ. Press, 2007.

———. *"My Madness Saved Me": The Madness and Marriage of Virginia Woolf.* New Brunswick, N.J.: Transaction Publishers, 2006.

———. "The Myth of Mental Illness." *American Psychologist* 15 (Feb. 1960): 113–18.

———. *The Myth of Mental Illness: Foundations of a Theory of Personal Conduct.* 1961. New York: HarperCollins, 1974.

———. *The Myth of Psychotherapy: Mental Healing as Religion, Rhetoric, and Repression.* 1978. Reprint, Syracuse: Syracuse Univ. Press, 1988.

———. *Pain and Pleasure: A Study of Bodily Feelings.* 2d ed. 1957. Reprint, Syracuse: Syracuse Univ. Press, 1988.

———. *Pharmacracy: Medicine and Politics in America.* 2001. Reprint, Syracuse: Syracuse Univ. Press, 2003.

———. *Psychiatric Justice.* 1965. Reprint, Syracuse: Syracuse Univ. Press, 1988.

———. *Psychiatric Slavery: When Confinement and Coercion Masquerade as Cure.* 1977. Reprint, Syracuse: Syracuse Univ. Press, 1989.

———. *Schizophrenia: The Sacred Symbol of Psychiatry.* 1976. Reprint, Syracuse: Syracuse Univ. Press, 1988.

———. *The Second Sin.* Garden City, N.Y.: Doubleday-Anchor, 1973.

———. *The Therapeutic State: Psychiatry in the Mirror of Current Events.* Buffalo: Prometheus Books, 1984.

———. *The Untamed Tongue: A Dissenting Dictionary.* LaSalle, Ill.: Open Court, 1990.

———. *Words to the Wise: A Medical-Philosophical Dictionary.* New Brunswick, N.J.: Transaction, 2003.

———, ed. *The Age of Madness: A History of Involuntary Mental Hospitalization Presented in Selected Texts.* Garden City, N.Y.: Doubleday-Anchor, 1973.

Thomas, K. *Religion and the Decline of Magic.* London: Weidenfeld and Nicolson, 1971.

Truzzi, Marcello. "Sherlock Holmes: Applied Social Scientist." In *The Sign of Three: Dupin, Holmes, Peirce,* edited by U. Eco and T. Sebeok, 55–80. Bloomington: Indiana Univ. Press, 1983.

Wasserstein, B. *The Secret Lives of Trebitsch Lincoln.* New Haven: Yale Univ. Press, 1988.

Wayland, F. *The Elements of Moral Science.* Edited by Joseph L. Blau. 1835. Cambridge: Harvard Univ. Press, 1963.

Webster, Brenda. *The Last Good Freudian.* New York: Holmes and Meier, 2000.

Wenegrad, Brant. *Theater of Disorder: Patients, Doctors, and the Construction of Illness.* Oxford: Oxford Univ. Press, 2001.

Wilbur, G. B., and W. Muensterberger, eds. *Psychoanalysis and Culture.* New York: International Universities Press, 1951.

Williams, Tennessee. *Memoirs.* New York: Bantam, 1976.

Wynne, F. *I Was Vermeer: The Legend of the Forger Who Swindled the Nazis.* London: Bloomsbury, 2006.

Yeo, Richard. *Defining Science: William Whewell, Natural Knowledge, and Public Debate in Victorian England.* Cambridge: Cambridge Univ. Press, 1993.

Young, Allan. *The Harmony of Illusions: Inventing Post-Traumatic Stress Disorder.* Princeton: Princeton Univ. Press, 1995.

Zweig, Stefan. *Mental Healers: Franz Anton Mesmer, Mary Baker Eddy, Sigmund Freud.* Translated by Eden Paul and Cedar Paul. 1932. Reprint, New York: Frederick Ungar, 1962.

———. "Portrait of Freud" (1932). In *Freud as We Knew Him,* edited by H. M. Ruitenbeek, 90–97. Detroit: Wayne State Univ. Press, 1973.

Index